HEALTH FOR THE PACIFIC 3

Common Diseases

in Papua New Guinea

compiled by Andrew Solien

OXFORD

Contents

Foreword

The lack of clear, simple and accurate information about good health contributes to poor health in any society.

The Health for the Pacific series is intended to educate and highlight important health issues that are affecting the lives of Papua New Guineans.

Common diseases such as malaria contribute to ill health. Therefore, there is a need to educate our people to be aware of their health, the risks to which they are exposed and the preventive measures that must be taken to combat diseases in order to lessen their impact in the communities, villages, towns and cities.

Health is everyone's concern.

I commend the compiler, Andrew Solien, Oxford University Press and the many others who have contributed to the publishing of these health books for schools in Papua New Guinea.

I trust that these books will play an important role in creating a healthy, strong and fit community for a better nation.

Dr Nicholas Mann CMS, MBBS, DCH, FACHSE

Acknowledgments

Papua New Guinea is a rich and diverse culture, with more than 700 languages spoken by its estimated 5.9 million people. It is the biggest island in the South Pacific, apart from Australia (which is also a continent) and Indonesia, with whom it shares its border.

This booklet is a compilation of resource materials written specifically for the education of students throughout Papua New Guinea, and for a variety of people in other institutions. Its aim is to provide education about the common diseases found throughout Papua New Guinea and to promote preventive health measures.

I would like to thank and acknowledge the National Department of Health—in particular, Dr Greg Law—for providing technical and other resource materials. I would also like to thank the many people whom I have interviewed while compiling this book. Their time and effort has been invaluable.

Lastly, I would like to thank Oxford University Press for recognising the need to publish health materials for schools in Papua New Guinea.

Andrew Solien

Chapter 1 The causes of disease

Every part of the body is made up of many small parts called cells. Cells of one kind can make up organs such as the liver, heart, lungs and so on. Together all the organs, bones and muscles make up a complete body.

Diseases cause illness (sickness) and suffering. They cause our bodies to stop working properly. Some can even cause death.

Diseases are not caused by accidents, but you could accidentally be exposed to a disease and become sick.

There are two main types of diseases: infectious diseases and non-infectious diseases.

Infectious diseases

Many organisms in the world are good for us. For example:

- ☑ Organisms break down dead animals and plant rubbish, and create rich, fertile soil.
- ☑ Some organisms in the mouth and intestine break down food and keep our bodies healthy.

But some common infectious diseases are spread through small living organisms that can harm us. Small animals (such as worms, insects, protozoa, fungi, bacteria and viruses) can invade our bodies and cause severe sickness.

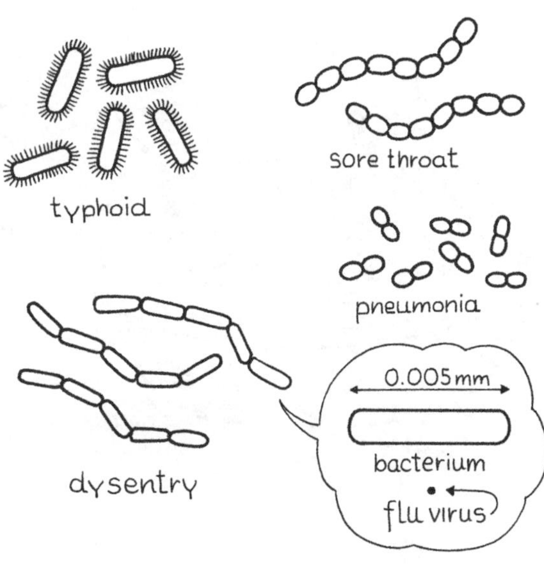

These organisms can enter the body:

- ☑ through the mouth with food and water
- ☑ through the nose or mouth when we breathe
- ☑ through cuts and sores in the skin
- ☑ by insect bites
- ☑ by contact from person to person.

Germs are very small living things that spread disease. Germs can only be seen through a microscope. We can prevent germs from spreading by:

- ☑ keeping our house and surroundings clean
- ☑ washing our body, clothes and bed linen regularly
- ☑ cleaning our teeth to prevent germs in the mouth

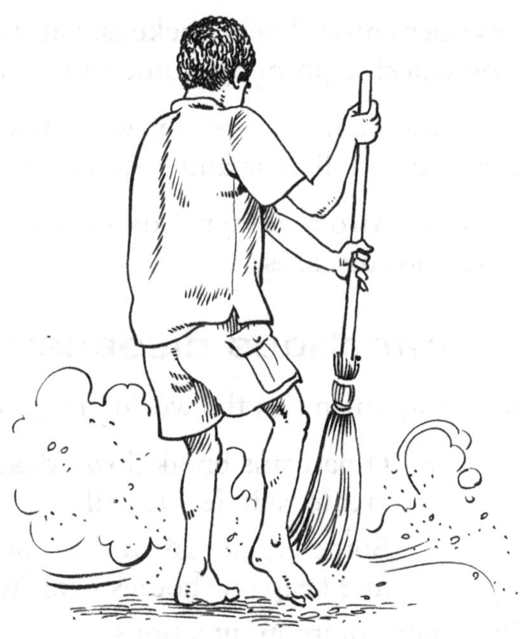

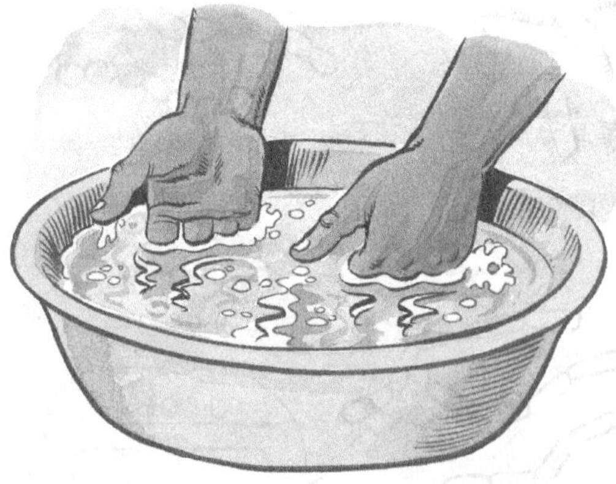

- ☑ covering food so that germ-carrying flies and other insects do not touch it
- ☑ washing our hands after going to the toilet
- ☑ washing our hands before preparing food.

The body naturally fights against infections. It can also be strengthened by immunisations (medicines that make the body immune to a particular disease). The medicines help the body to produce antibodies. The antibodies fight against diseases such as whooping cough, polio and so on.

Immunisation can protect us from some diseases by putting certain substances into our body that will protect us. This substance is usually injected with a needle.

In PNG, it does not cost you any money to be immunised against some diseases by a health worker. The vaccine must be given at the right age and for the right number of doses.

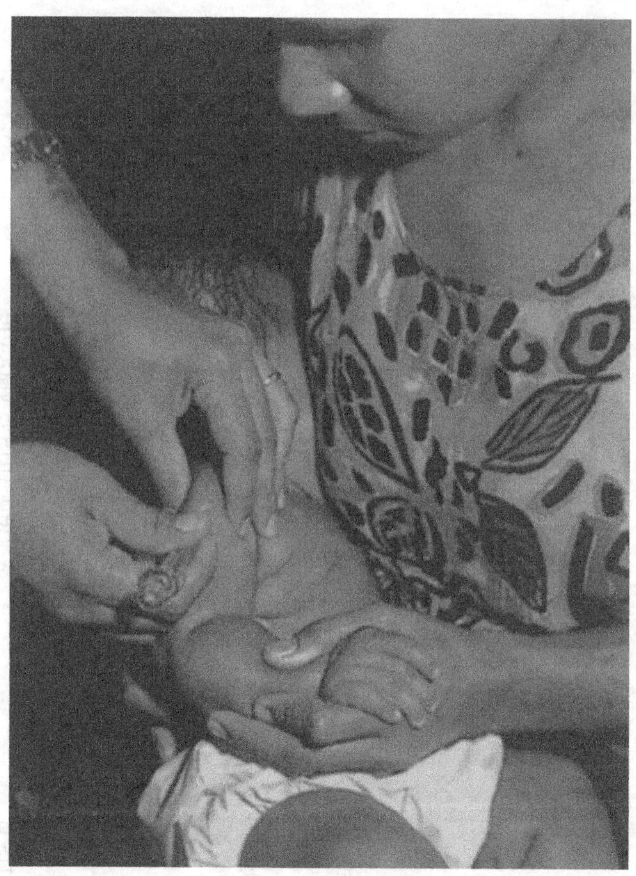

Disease	Vaccine	How many doses?	When are the doses given?
Whooping cough, diphtheria, tetanus	Triple antigen	3	**1** When the child is one month old **2** One month after first dose **3** One month after second dose
Pigpel	Pigbel	5	**1** When the child is one month old **2** One month after first dose **3** One month after second dose **4** First year of elementary school **5** Last year of elementary school
Measles	Measles	2	**1** When the child is six months old **2** Three months after first dose
Poliomyelitis	Sabin oral vaccine	4	**1** As soon as possible after birth **2** At one month of age **3** One month after second dose **4** One month after third dose
Tuberculosis	BCG vaccine	1	As soon as possible after birth
Hepatitis B	Hepatitis B vaccine	3	**1** As soon as possible after birth **2** At least one month after first dose **3** At least two months after second dose
Tetanus toxoid	Tetanus	2	**1** First year of elementary school **2** Last year of elementary school

Activity 1·1

Read the immunisation chart on page 4 and answer the following questions.

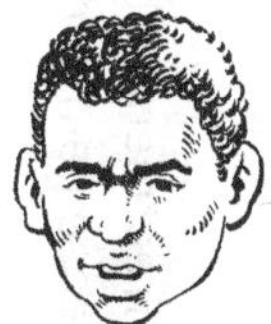

1. Why are children given vaccines at such an early age?
2. Why do you think some children are not immunised?
3. What happens to children who are not immunised?

Non-infectious diseases

A non-infectious disease is one that does not spread from person to person. There are different causes of non-infectious diseases in the body:

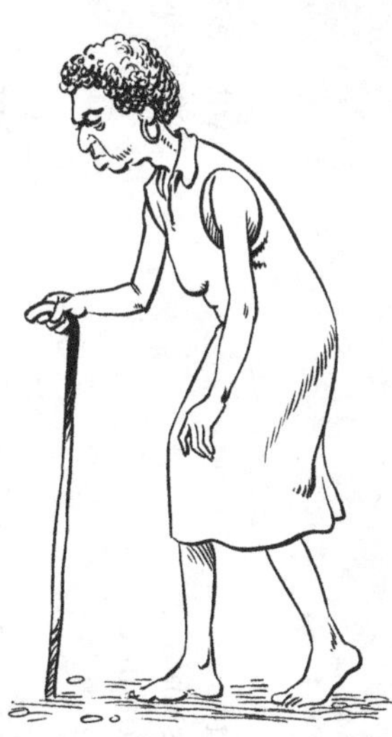

- Some problems are caused by the body itself. Body parts get old and wear out. Arthritis (problems with joints) and cataracts (difficulty with eyes, blurred vision) are common as we grow older. Some body parts grow too fast and take over the body (cancer). This can happen at any age.
- Other problems come from outside the body. Poisons can come from different sources: smoking and industrial poisons (from factories) can make people very sick.
- Not eating right can also make people very sick. If we eat too much fat and sugar, and drink too much alcohol, our bodies can become diseased. Lack of something the body needs can cause diseases such as malnutrition, goitre (swelling of the neck) and scurvy (disease cause by lack of Vitamin C).

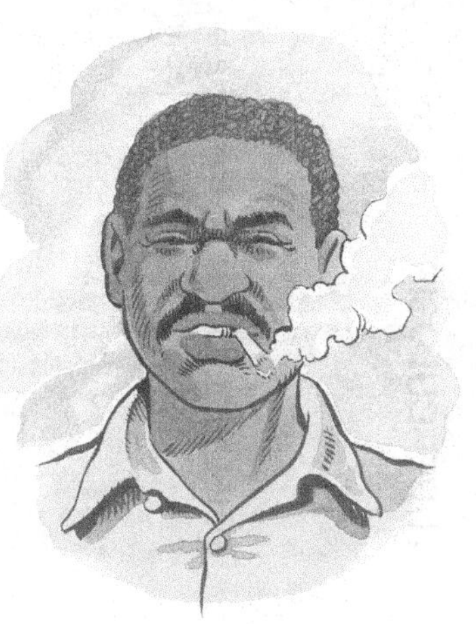

Main infectious diseases in Papua New Guinea

Disease	How do I get infected?	How does it spread?	What medicine do I need to take?	How can I use water to treat or prevent the disease?
MALARIA	A mosquito bites through your skin and injects protozoa into your bloodstream	Blood	Antimalarial medicines	Treatment: Drink plenty of water and other liquids.
TYPHOID	Typhoid bacteria are ingested (taken in by mouth with food or drink)	• Flies • Food and water • Contact with faeces	Antibiotic medicine	Prevention: • Boil all drinking water to kill bacteria • Wash hands after using toilet, before preparing food and before eating Treatment: Drinks lots of water to prevent dehydration
TUBERCULOSIS	Bacteria are breathed in	• Coughing • Spitting • Sneezing	Anti-TB medicines Antibiotics used together	Treatment: • Drinks lots of water • Breathe steam to loosen mucus
PNEUMONIA	Bacteria are breathed in	Air	Antibiotics	Treatment: • Drinks lots of water • Breathe steam to loosen mucus
MEASLES & CHICKEN POX	Virus is spread by inhalation or contact with infected people or things	Droplets in air	Paracetemol for fever and pain Vaccinations can help prevent the disease	Treatment: Cold compresses to ease pain and itching

DIARRHOEA	Virus or bacteria are ingested through food or water	• Flies • Food and water	Paracetemol for fever and pain	Prevention: • Boil drinking water • Wash hands after using toilet, before preparing food and before eating Treatment: Drink lots of water to prevent dyhydration
INFECTED SORE AND WOUNDS	Bacteria get into open wounds	• Contact with dirty objects • Flies	Antibiotics	Treatment: • Wash wounds often, using soap • Soak infected area in hot water or use compresses
SEXUALLY TRANSMITTED INFECTIONS (GONORRHOEA, SYPHILIS)	Viruses are passed between people when they have sex	• Sexual activity without using condoms • Contact with discharges (pus, liquids) from sores	Antibiotics	Treatment: Drink lots of water
COLDS, INFLUENZA	Virus is breathed in	Droplets in air	Paracetamol for fever and pain	Treatment: • For high fever, soak body in cool water • Drink lots of water
AIDS	Viruses are passed between people when they have sex	• Sexual activity without using condoms • Contact with discharges (pus, liquids) from sores	Paracetamol for fever There is no cure	Treatment: Drink lots of water

How to take care of a sick person

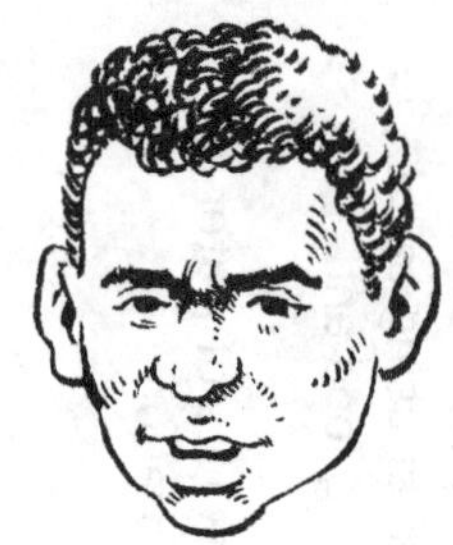

Always seek help at the first sign of a dangerous illness. Do not wait until people are so ill that it becomes impossible to take them to a health centre or hospital.

Sickness weakens the body. To gain strength and get well quickly, people need special care. The following are the basic things to do to care for sick people:

- ☑ Make sure sick people are comfortable and resting in a quiet place with plenty of fresh air and light. They should be kept from getting too hot or cold.
- ☑ Give sick people plenty to drink. In nearly every sickness the body needs plenty of liquids such as water, tea or juice, but not alcohol.
- ☑ Make sure sick people have healthy food. Sick people need a lot of fluids and need to eat nourishing foods such as chicken, eggs, fish, green vegetables and fruit. Energy foods such as sweet potato, cassava and rice are also important.
- ☑ Sick people need to be clean. They should be bathed each day. If they are too sick to get out of bed, wash them with a sponge or cloth and lukewarm water. Sheets and covers must also be clean to prevent diseases from spreading.

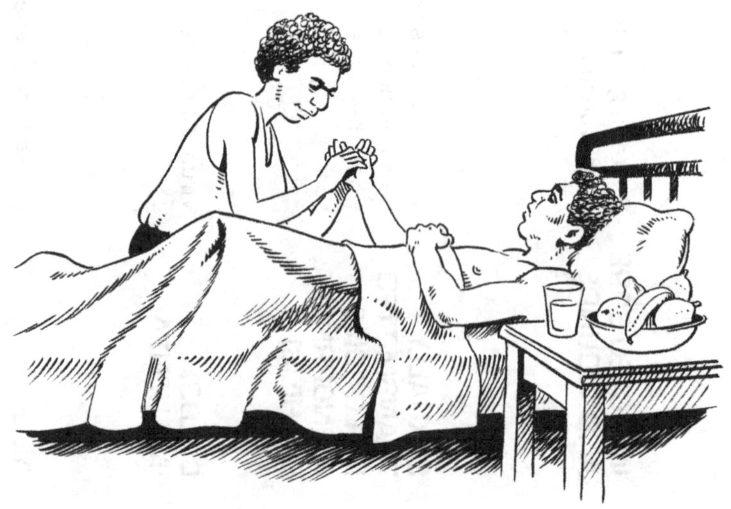

Chapter 2 Malaria and other diseases carried by mosquitoes

 Malaria

Malaria is a serious disease that is sometimes fatal. It is caused by malaria parasites (small organism) entering a person's bloodstream.

People of all ages can get malaria. It is most dangerous for babies, young children and pregnant women.

When a mosquito bites a person, it puts the parasites into the person's body. The parasites then destroy the red blood cells in the body, which causes sickness.

If a mosquito that carries malaria parasites bites a person who does not have malaria, the malaria parasite will move from the person to the mosquito. In this way, malaria becomes very widespread.

You do not get malaria by drinking water or eating food where mosquitoes have laid their eggs.

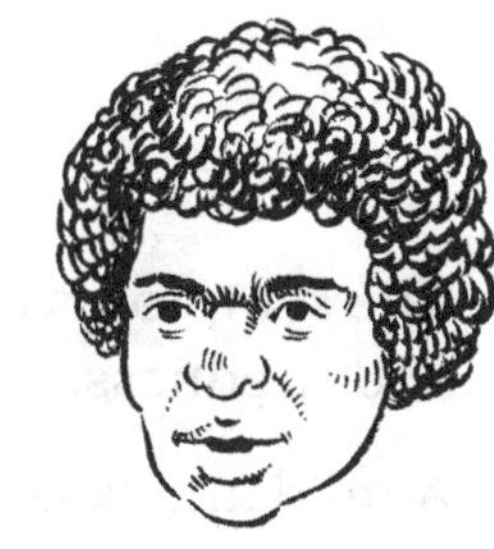

Malaria is contracted from the bite of an infected female anopheline mosquito. This female anopheline mosquito bites mostly at night and feeds on blood to reproduce her young.

The malaria mosquito can be recognised by its resting position: its tail points upwards when it is biting or resting.

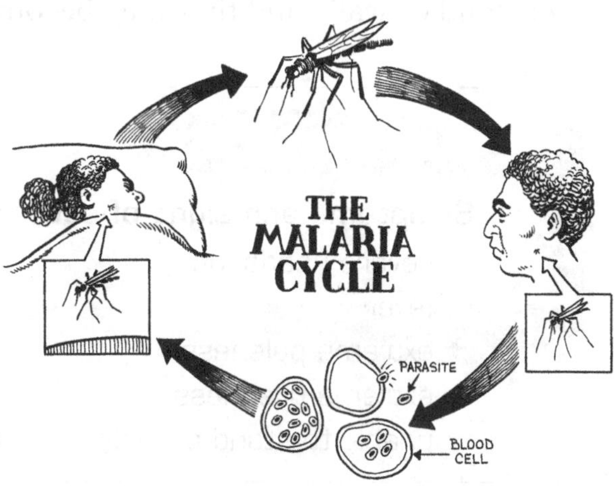

What are the symptoms of malaria?

People who have malaria have a fever, their bodies get hot and cold, they have aching muscles or joints and sometimes headaches. Malaria attacks can be mild or severe (very serious).

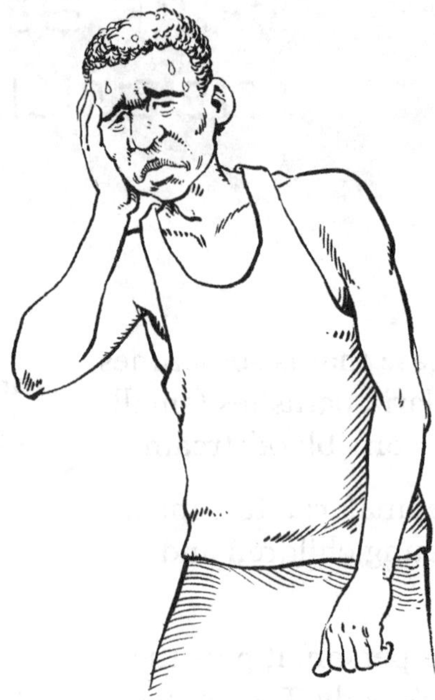

The symptoms and signs of mild malaria are headache, fever, paleness and tiredness.

A mild attack of malaria can be present in people's bodies without the people being very sick.

Severe malaria can make people very sick. People may be so sick that they cannot stand or walk, and they may become unconscious.

INFORMATION

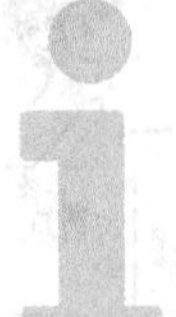

Symptoms and signs of severe malaria:

- severe headache
- fever
- extreme paleness
- extreme tiredness
- unable to stand or walk
- vomiting or severe diarrhoea
- unusual behaviour
- fits or convulsions
- unconsciousness.

What is the treatment for malaria?

Antimalarials are special medicines used to kill the malaria parasite. The health worker at the Aid Post or Health Centre will prescribe the right type of tablets and the correct dosage you need to take.

For severe malaria the treatment will be carried out in an Aid Post or Health Centre. The treatment involves:

- ☑ taking a blood sample from the patient
- ☑ treating the patient with the correct drugs.

You should come back to the Aid Post if there is no improvement and the symptoms continue.

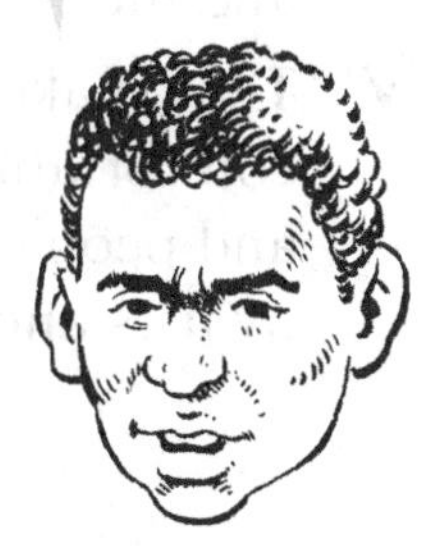

How can malaria be prevented?

We can prevent people getting malaria by:

- ☑ killing mosquitoes
- ☑ stopping mosquitoes from biting people, such as by using treated mosquito nets
- ☑ stopping mosquitoes from multiplying by getting rid of water they breed in
- ☑ giving people medicines that will kill the malaria parasites that are in their bodies.
- ☑ Using coils and repellents to keep mosquitoes away.

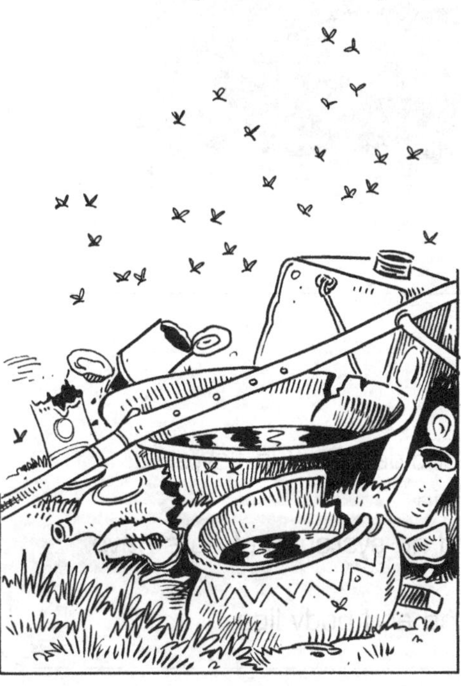

- ☑ Use permethrin-treated bed nets to kill mosquitoes and other insects too. Dry treated bed nets are safe. The nets must be clean and dry. They must also be without holes so that mosquitoes cannot enter the bed area while people are asleep. Treated bed nets are available at cost through Rotary Against Malaria and the National Department of Health.
- ☑ Cut the grass and clean around the house and surroundings. Burn rubbish and bury tins and shells. This will make the area less attractive to mosquitoes.

Treated bed nets

Although the use of treated bed nets has helped control the rise in malaria sickness, many people are concerned about the use of treated bed nets.

- ☑ They stop mosquitoes from biting and spreading sickness.
- ☑ They keep away mosquitoes and flies.
- ☑ They make sleeping more comfortable: the air is warm and people are not disturbed by flies and mosquitoes.

- ☒ With both treated and untreated nets, people feel hot and uncomfortable inside a net, complaining of a lack of circulating air.
- ☒ People complain of lack of space to move.
- ☒ Treated nets smell, particularly when they are first treated.
- ☒ They are expensive.

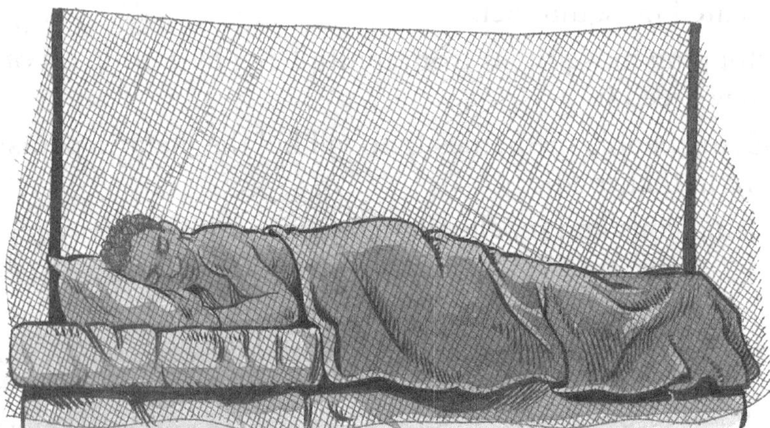

INFORMATION

Permethrin

→ Permethrin is a natural insecticide found in flowers.

→ Treat bed nets with permethrin.

→ It is non-toxic to humans, and no systemic effects have been reported.

→ Use it as a treatment for head and body lice.

The fight against malaria

Malaria is the leading cause of admissions to health facilities in PNG, according to Dr Nicholas Mann, the Secretary for Health. In an interview for a health radio program he said, 'malaria is related to mosquitoes, and mosquitoes are related to water where their eggs flourish'. He also said that mosquitoes breed during the wet season, and advises children and old people to take antimalaria medicine and use bed nets to avoid becoming sick.

He said that the 2001–2010 National Health Plan of the National Department of Health has made malaria a priority. Its objective is to halve the number of malarial deaths and sickness, and to make treatment available in areas where malaria is common [by 2005].

The Department, in its **Roll Back Malaria** program, made it a priority to promote treated mosquito bed nets to control malaria control in PNG.

Between 1995 and 1997, 642 people were reported to have died because of malaria and there was a total of 32 046 out patients admitted to hospital with malaria in PNG.

To fight against malaria, the National Department of Health wants to make sure that people are diagnosed quickly and given the proper treatment.

House spraying is also important in areas where malaria is very common, which is mainly in the highlands. It is also important to drain excess water around people's homes, and not to leave water standing in large containers or puddles.

The National Health Department also wants 80 to 100 per cent of the population using treated bed nets. The Secretary for Health also said that bed nets should not be washed, but should be re-treated every six months. He advised that health officers in the Provinces will help re-treat and distribute treated bed nets.

Activity 2·1 *Community awareness*

It is important that your community fight actively against malaria. This can be done by:

- cleaning the puddles where mosquitoes breed
- cutting grass and flowers short so that mosquitoes don't have a place to live
- throwing away old tyres, tins and coconut shells where water can collect.

You can help personally by:

- encouraging your family and friends to clean around their yards to control mosquitoes
- encouraging such things as using treated bed nets, and screening windows and doors
- encouraging people who think they have malaria to go to the clinic for treatment.

Activity 2·2 *Group activity*

Singing is an art. It gives people a chance to show their feelings and share their hopes by giving a message to an audience.

In this activity, small groups will express their feelings about malaria by writing a song. After you have written the words, choose music to go with them. When you have completed the song, present it in a booklet so that others can read it.

The main points you should deal with are:

- what malaria is
- how you get malaria
- where you can be treated if you have malaria
- what you can do to stop malaria.

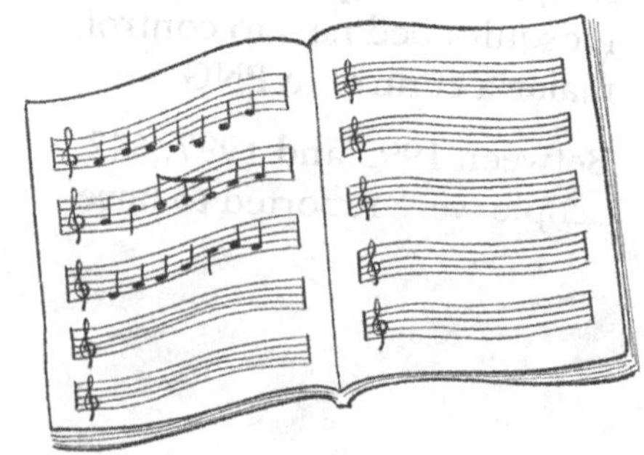

You are encouraged to write in your own tok ples or mother tongue, rather than Pidgin, English or Motu.

Activity 2·3 *Ann*

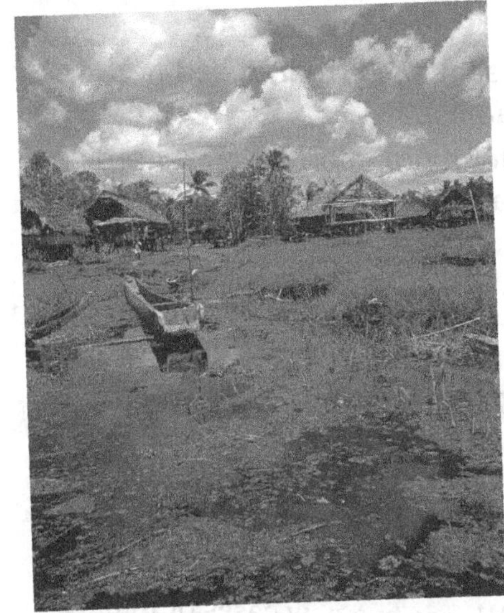

Ann lives in a small village in the highlands. It is the rainy season. The grass has grown fast and the small puddles of water are everywhere. To make matters worse, there are a lot of mosquitoes biting, too!

On her way past the village Aid Post to the river, Ann has seen a lot of mothers with their children lining up to be treated for malaria. She laughs at them, and says to herself, 'I won't get sick from malaria. I don't spend a lot of time with dirty people!'

After reading about Ann, answer the following questions:

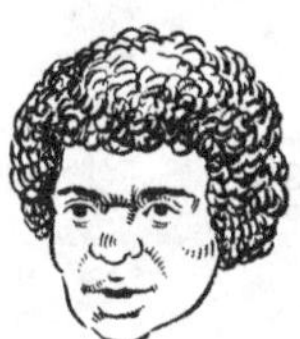

1 What do you think about Ann's belief that she won't get malaria?

2 What would you do if you were in her place?

Activity 2·4 *Bed nets*

The National Health Department, as part of its Roll Back Malaria program, has sent health workers to your village. They have been told to help the village people have their mosquito nets retreated with permethrin.

At the village, the health workers find out that some of the villagers have been washing their treated bed nets upstream. Other villagers have been using the nets to kill head lice.

After reading about the bed nets, answer the following questions:

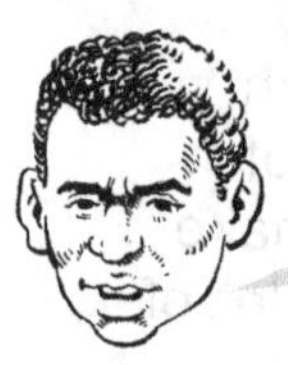

1. Do you think that washing your treated bed nets upstream is wise?
2. What is your opinion about the treated bed nets being used to kill head lice?
3. Who should you see for more information regarding the proper use of treated bed nets?

Veifa'a

In the fight against malarial deaths in the rural areas of PNG, we go on a trip to Veifa'a village in the Central Province to see how the youths are trained to carry out awareness on malaria.

It is dry and dusty all around. The water level of rivers along the highway was very low, some rivers were entirely dry. But the mosquitoes were twice as big and sucking painfully on our skin for blood.

This is Veifa'a home in the Bereina district. It is also where the Mekeos, Kairukus and many other tribes live too.

Our purpose was mainly to find out the progress of the malaria workshop in Central Province.

It was around 5:00 pm when we arrived at the village. We were brought to the nursing school where we were to board and lodge for the night. Sooner than expected, I bumped into the Head Sister, Rose Awae, and it was like old friends talking.

'We see five new cases of malaria each day, and we admit two or three people to the health centre. But we do not have a malaria laboratory so we treat people on the basis of their symptoms. If there is no response to the treatment, we have to send patients to Port Moresby for tests and treatment.'

'When people get malaria,' she added, 'they blame sorcery.'

Sister Awae's account of her experiences with the village people does not surprise me. Even in the urban centres and cities where medical services are available, people, regardless of the cause and symptoms of malaria, tend to believe in black magic or some kind of traditional link to its cause.

→

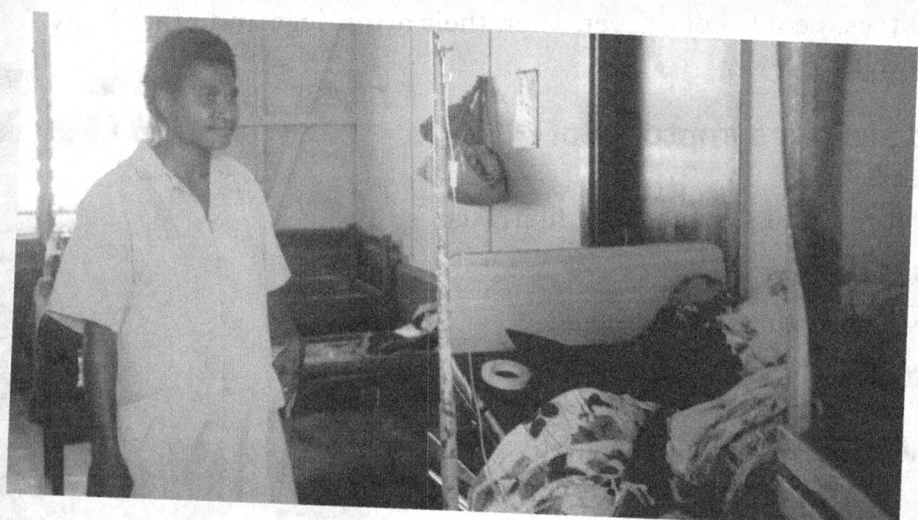

Such attitudes have made it difficult for health workers to communicate with people. Health workers now involve the people in drama to educate them about malaria and how best to fight it.

In the morning, I see youths preparing the malaria workshop drama for presentation.

'The main aim of the workshop is to get the message across to the community. We want to improve people's lives and try to prevent diseases coming into the community,' said James Aisa, who is in charge of the drama workshop here.

Everyone at the workshop had a say about malaria and the drama was received well by all present. This was the purpose of the drama workshop: to help people to fight against malaria and give them control over their own health and lives.

Despite the dirt and dust in the area, we were pleased to see such a positive attitude in the community. People were responding to health workers, taking charge of their own lives and making a real effort to fight against malaria in their village.

I said to myself that if only such programs as this reached all people in the rural areas of PNG, malaria would disappear. This may seem like a dream, but you never know what to expect in the land of the unexpected. Only time will tell.

Filariasis

Filariasis is a disease caused by the mosquito. After being bitten by mosquitoes, people get a fever. Then their arms, legs and other body parts swell.

What are the symptoms of filariasis?

There are several symptoms of filariasis:

- fever
- sometimes chills
- pain and swelling of lymph glands and groin
- in severe cases, swelling of whole arm or leg or scrotum or breast
- in severe cases, the skin is thick and hard.

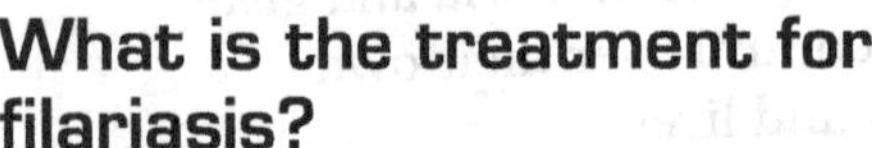

What is the treatment for filariasis?

If you have these symptoms and think you might have filariasis, go to the hospital for a check-up and treatment.

- Medicines can be given for this disease.
- A crepe bandage can be applied to the arm or leg to stop swelling.
- In severe cases some surgery may be needed.

How can filariasis be prevented?

We can prevent people getting filariasis by:

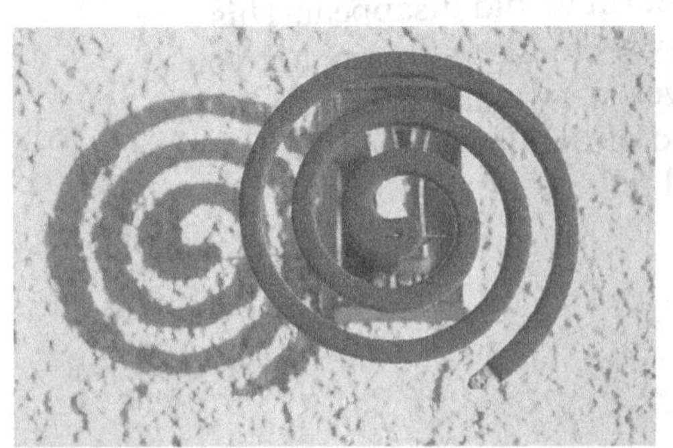

- spraying inside walls with an insecticide, installing fly screens in houses, and using bed nets and insect repellents
- eliminating breeding places, such as open toilets, old tyres, etc.
- clearing ponds of vegetation, and applying herbicides to plants where mosquitoes breed.

Chapter 3 Acute Respiratory Infection (ARI)

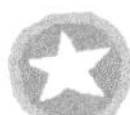 ARI

ARI is the abbreviation (short form) of Acute Respiratory Infection. These are the most common diseases causing serious health problems to the people of PNG. ARIs affect the respiratory tract. They are generally spread by coughing, sneezing and talking.

ARIs are infections that almost always start with a cough over a period of a few days or weeks. There are a few symptoms of ARI, as shown at right.

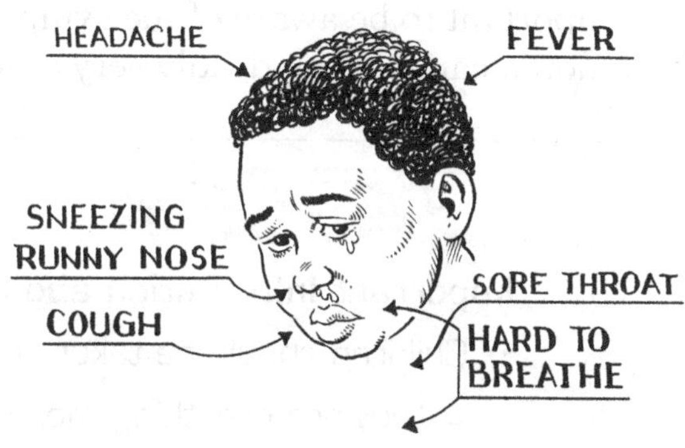

Coughing is a typical sign of any infection of the respiratory tract. The main difference is the duration of cough. Since coughing is a common symptom in many ARIs, it is important to find out what kind of ARI you have.

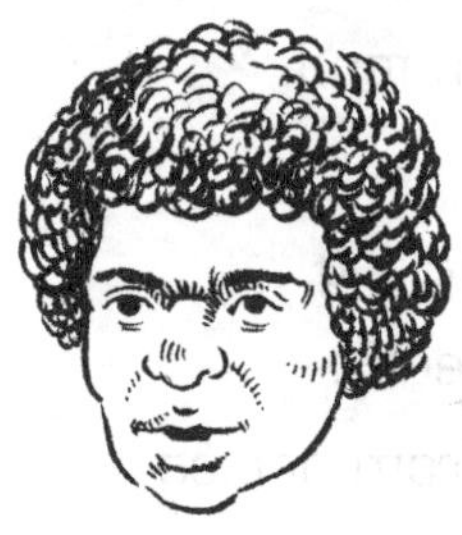

If you have cough that lasts a long time, go to a Health Centre for advice or treatment.

Many children in PNG die from ARI. Lung infection (pneumonia) is one kind of ARI and is the biggest cause of death in PNG. It is especially bad for children under 7 years of age. There are also other kinds of ARI. We will look at them in detail next.

Pneumonia

This is a very common infection. It is the biggest killer of young children in PNG. It often occurs after a cold or influenza.

What are the symptoms of pneumonia?

- ☑ cough
- ☑ fever
- ☑ fast, shallow breathing
- ☑ restlessness
- ☑ blue around the mouth
- ☑ poor appetite.

What is the treatment for pneumonia?

People with pneumonia die quickly if they are not given antibiotics, such as penicillin and amoxicillin, at a health centre or Aid Post.

It is important to be aware of the symptoms so that you can act quickly. Pneumonia can become deadly very quickly!

INFORMATION

Important Information about pneumonia!

→ Children should be taken to an Aid Post or Health Centre if:

- they are breathing more rapidly than normal
- the lower part of the rib cage goes in as the child breathes in instead of going out as usual
- the child is unable to drink.

→ Encourage children to drink water and take in food.

→ Keep children warm but not hot.

→ Keep children away from cooking fires or smoking.

→ Help children breathe by clearing the nose gently.

→ Keep children and adults with coughs away from babies who can easily catch this disease.

Whooping cough

Whooping cough (pronounced 'hooping') is a serious, highly contagious disease of the respiratory system. It is a disease that is caused by bacteria. It is found all over the world, mostly among infants and young children.

The name whooping cough comes from the high-pitched whooping noise children make when they try to catch their breath after severe coughing attacks.

What are the symptoms of whooping cough?

Stage 1: Symptoms are like those of the common cold. Children have trouble breathing. They also cough and have a fever. This stage lasts from one to two weeks. The disease is very contagious at this time. It spreads through the spray of bacteria-filled droplets from the child's nose and mouth.

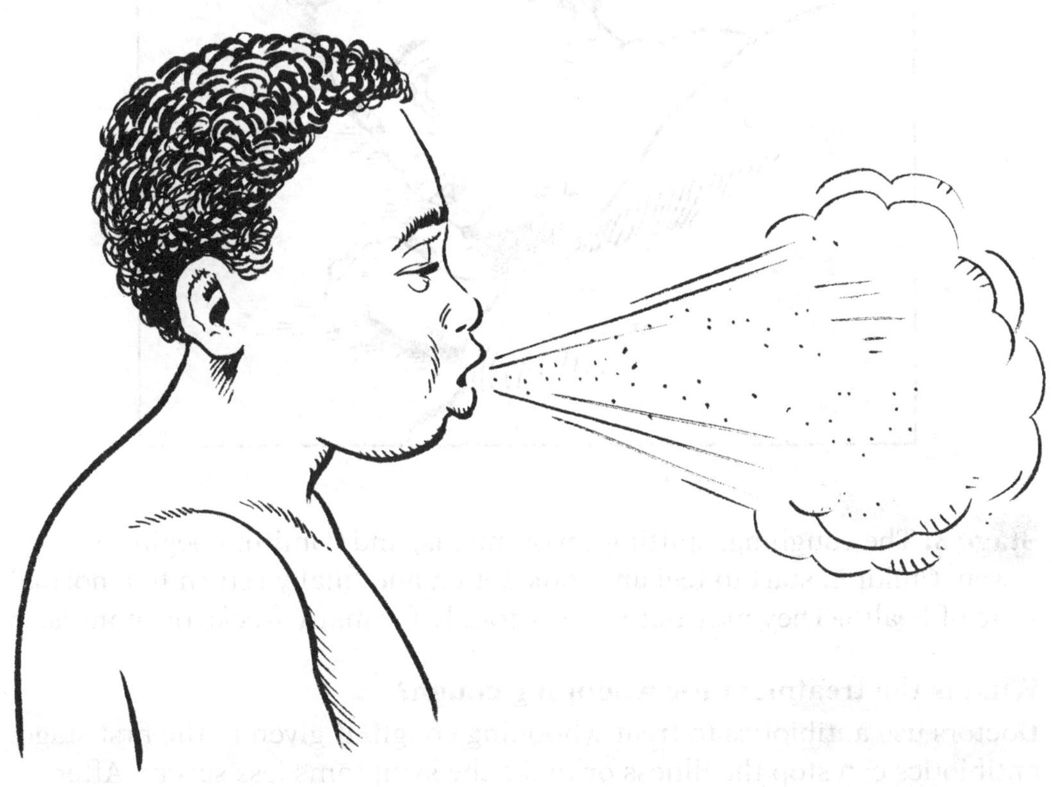

Stage 2: This is the most serious phase of the disease. It usually lasts from two to three weeks. The child will start coughing at night. Later, the child will cough both night and day, and will often spit up thick mucus after coughing. Infants often swallow the mucus and then vomit, which can cause them to become dehydrated (lose body water) and lose weight. Children can get pneumonia or their lungs can collapse. Children, especially infants under six months of age, may die during this stage.

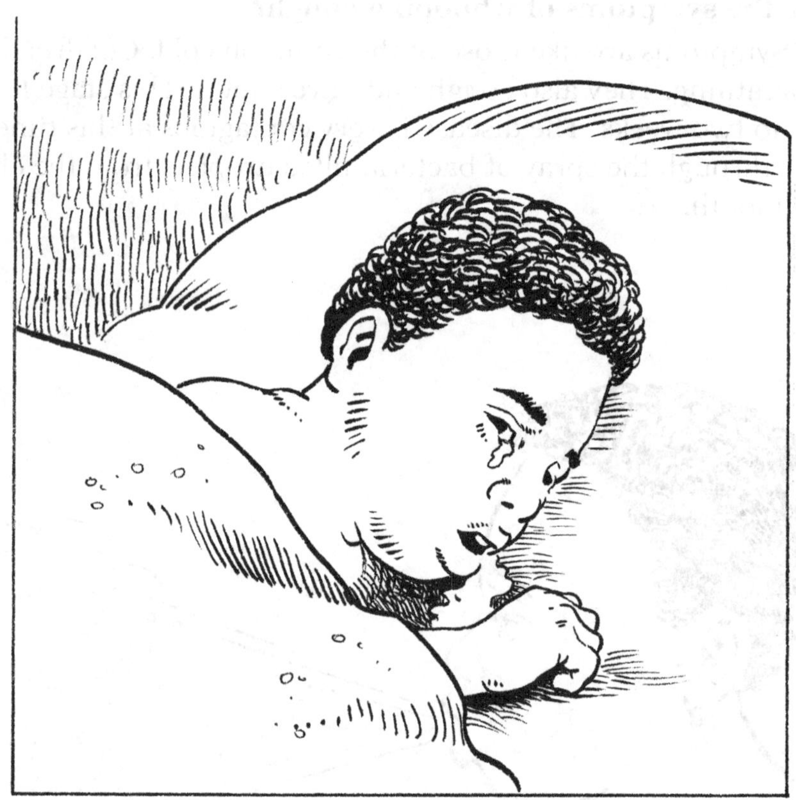

Stage 3: The coughing, spitting up of mucus, and vomiting begin to lessen. Children start to feel and look better, and finally return to a normal state of health. They may not recover totally for many weeks or months.

What is the treatment for whooping cough?

Doctors use antibiotics to treat whooping cough. If given in the first stage, antibiotics can stop the illness or make the symptoms less severe. After the second stage begins, major treatment involves helping the patient breathe freely and limiting the number of severe coughing attacks.

If you or any of your family members have the signs and symptoms of whooping cough as described in this section, go to the nearest clinic or hospital for treatment. Early treatment is very important.

Whooping cough is preventable. Babies and young children can be immunised with a vaccine to protect them.

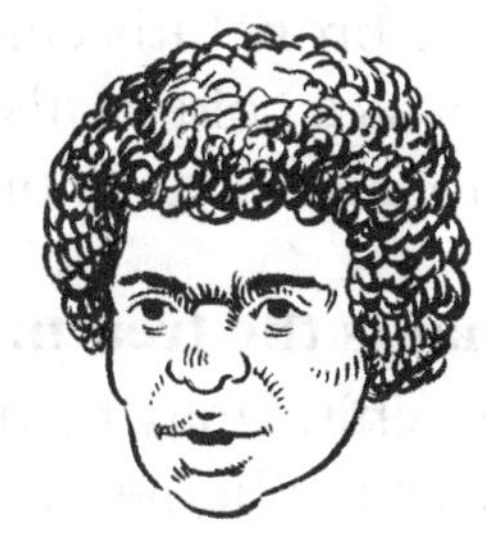

Bronchitis

Bronchitis (pronounced 'bronkaitis') is an inflammation of the lining of the air passages in the lungs. The inflammation causes these passages to produce more mucus, which is then coughed up. Bronchitis may be either acute (short-term and severe) or chronic (long lasting).

The structure of the lungs

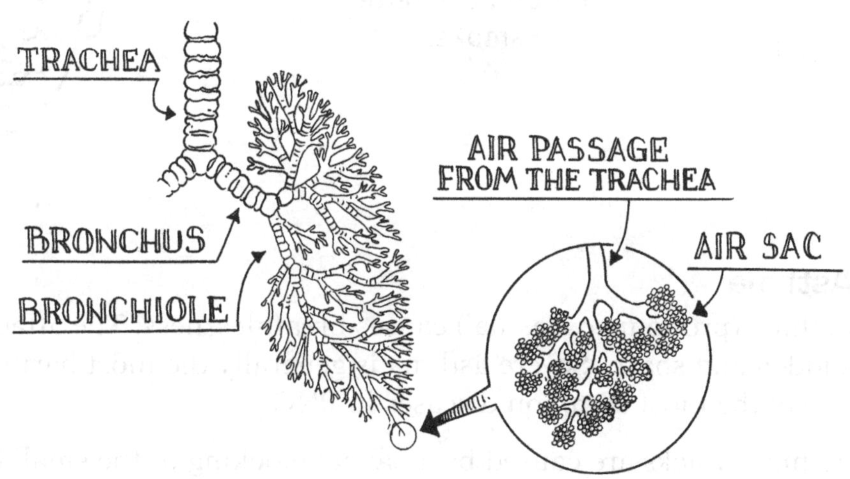

What are the symptoms of bronchitis?

People who have bronchitis have high fevers and chest pain. The also cough and bring up mucus.

Doctors consider the condition chronic if the coughing lasts for several months. Chronic bronchitis may produce shortness of breath. In very bad cases it can cause heart failure. The most common cause of chronic bronchitis is cigarette smoking. Either type of bronchitis may lead to asthma or pneumonia.

Acute bronchitis can be caused by a respiratory infection (lung infection), such as a cold. It also can be caused by breathing irritating fumes, such as tobacco smoke or polluted air.

What is the treatment for bronchitis?

Bronchitis may be treated with drugs that widen the bronchial tubes, or with a medicine that will loosen mucus so it can be coughed up more easily. Antibiotics are prescribed if a bacterial infection is present. Most cases of acute bronchitis clear up within weeks.

Moist air produced by steam also helps loosen mucus.

Chronic bronchitis cannot be cured, so it is especially important to avoid polluted air and cigarette smoke.

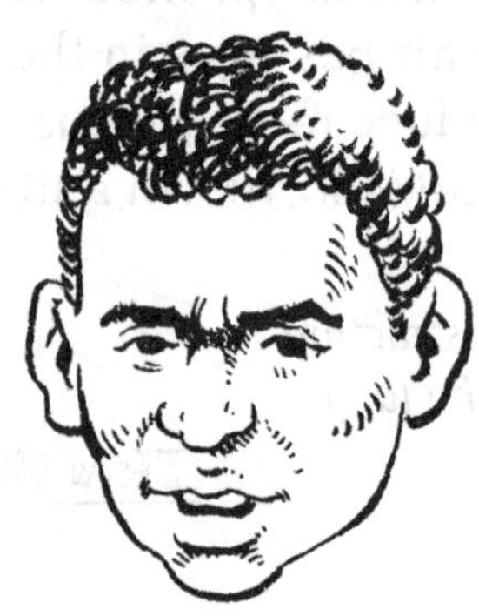

Asthma

Asthma (pronounced 'asma') causes breathlessness. The attacks can be sudden and sharp. Severe asthma is generally the most harmful and is one of the most common diseases in PNG.

Asthma attacks are caused by a partial blocking of the small bronchial tubes in the lungs. The most common kind of asthma is caused by a specific allergic reaction. In most cases, the allergy is caused by irritating substances, such as house dust, airborne pollens or certain foods.

Attacks of asthma often follow periods of heavy work or emotional strain. An infection of the nose and throat can cause the start of an attack. A sudden change in the weather may also bring on an attack. Asthma may occur at certain times of the year if the air contains specific pollens.

What are the symptoms of asthma?

Symptoms include a wheezing or whistling sound from the chest when breathing in, and even greater wheezing when breathing out. People with asthma may gasp for air and feel that they are suffocating.

When an attack of asthma begins, the person complains frequently of a feeling of tightness in the chest. The person has a hacking cough and is short of breath. Thick mucus develops in the lungs, and the cough becomes more intense. The person may feel better temporarily after coughing up the mucus.

What is the treatment for asthma?

Avoiding the things that cause asthma is the first step in treating asthma. A doctor will be able to offer a diagnosis and then prescribe the correct treatment. This may mean the asthmatic person will stop eating certain foods or doing certain kinds of activities.

Once an asthma attack starts, drugs that are inhaled (breathed in) can help make breathing easier.

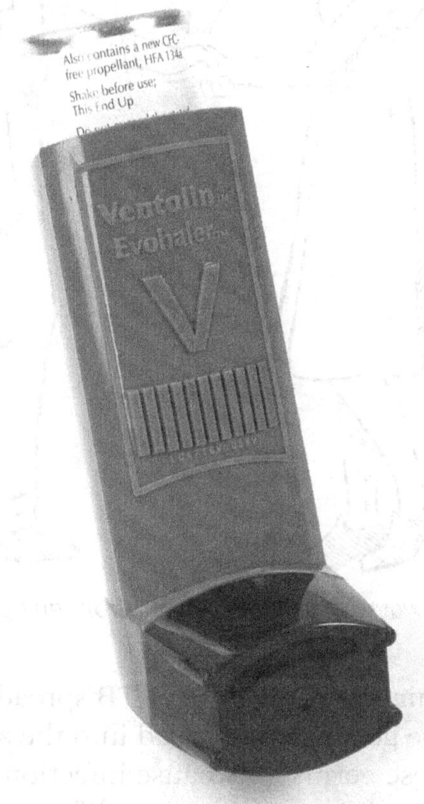

Tuberculosis (TB)

Tuberculosis (TB) is a major health concern in Papua New Guinea. It is a deadly infectious disease caused by the TB germ. It usually attacks the lungs and causes cavities (spaces) in the lungs. It is very contagious. This means it spreads easily from one person to another, so care must be taken to prevent its spread.

TB is a very serious problem. Without treatment, 50 per cent of people infected in PNG would die in five years. It is very important to be aware of the dangers of TB and the many ways people can catch it.

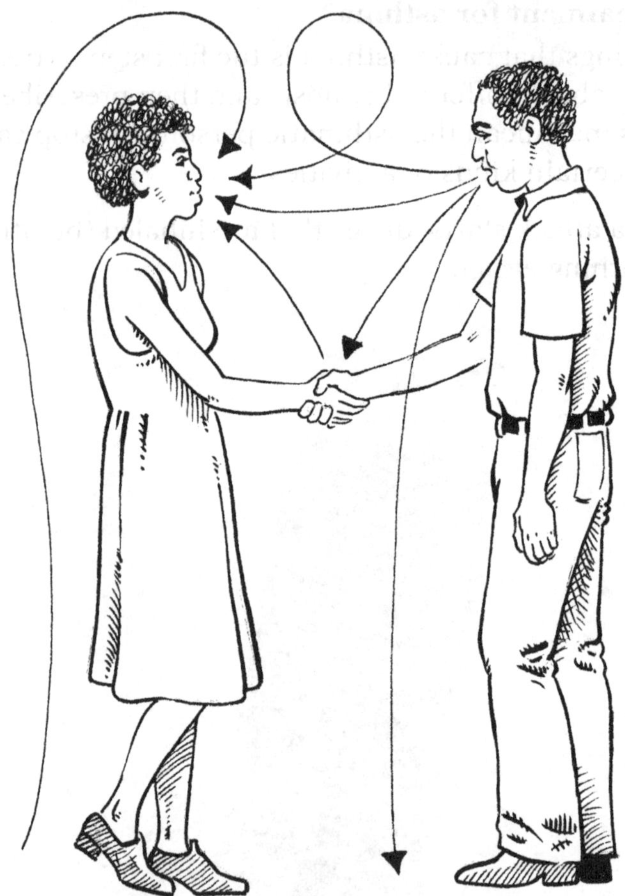

TB can be spread in many ways. It is easily passed from one person to another

TB is spread through air. People who have TB spread it when they cough, sneeze, spit or talk. The germs are released into the air and are breathed in by other people. These germs may cause infection. A single breath containing TB germs can infect someone for life.

If you take care of yourself, your body can fight the TB germs. Your defence (immune) system can overpower the TB germs from multiplying enough to cause illness.

But if the body defences are weak, the TB germs will invade your immune system and spread to other places, where they multiply.

What are the symptoms of TB?

The signs of TB include:

- ☑ coughing
- ☑ weight loss
- ☑ chest pain
- ☑ shortness of breath
- ☑ fever
- ☑ tiredness.

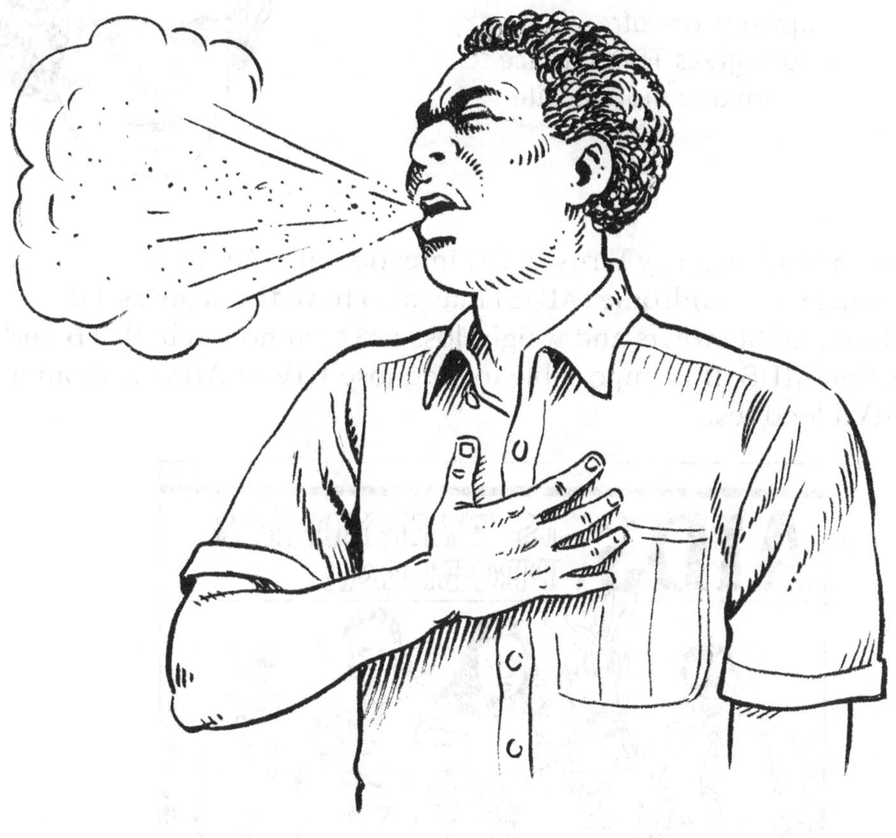

Coughing may go for weeks and you may cough up blood. The main difference between TB and other ARIs is the duration of the cough. If you cough for a long time and your situation gets worse, see a health worker to make sure you do not have TB.

When the TB germs enter the lungs, you may not know it. Some of the germs may be beaten by your body's natural defences, but some germs can remain dormant ('asleep') without your knowing. If the body's defences cannot fight against the TB germ, your body will become infected.

HIV-positive people can get TB easily. Their immune systems are already weak, so it gives TB a chance to invade more easily.

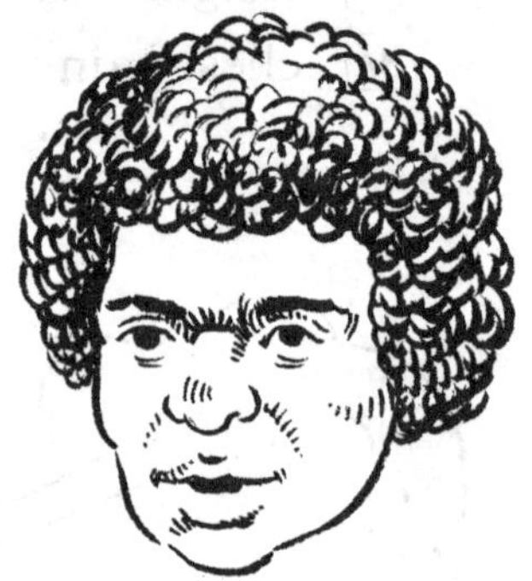

Human Immunodeficiency Virus (HIV) infection and Acquired Immunodeficiency Syndrome (AIDS) may also have the signs as TB. Fatigue, fever, night sweats and weight loss are common to both TB and HIV infection/AIDS. It is impossible to diagnose HIV or AIDS without a special HIV blood test.

AIDS IS EVERYONE'S PROBLEM!
A PERSON WITH AIDS IS JUST LIKE YOU AND ME.

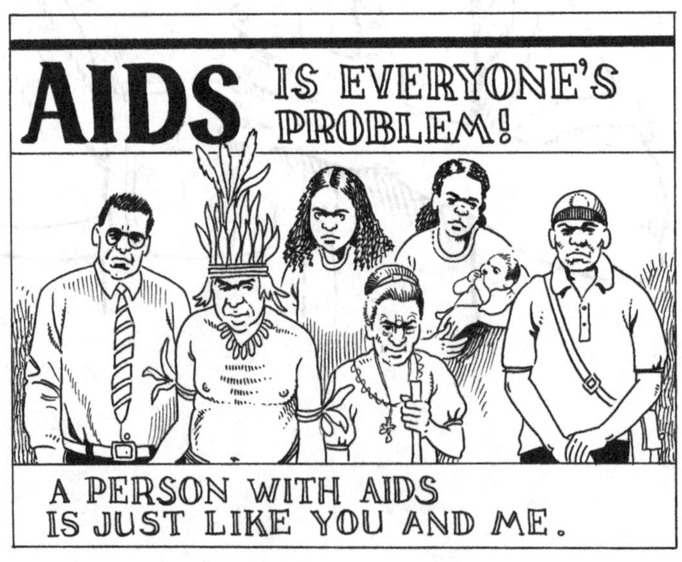

What is the treatment for TB?

If you have the symptoms of TB, see your health worker immediately. TB is a deadly and highly contagious disease, but it can be cured. If untreated, TB can kill.

The only way to find out whether if you have TB is by going to the hospital for a check-up. Three samples of your sputum (mucus in your spit) must be taken and examined at different times under a microscope. If the sputum contains TB germs, it means you are sick and infectious.

If this test is negative your chest may be X-rayed to determine whether you have changes in your lungs that might indicate TB.

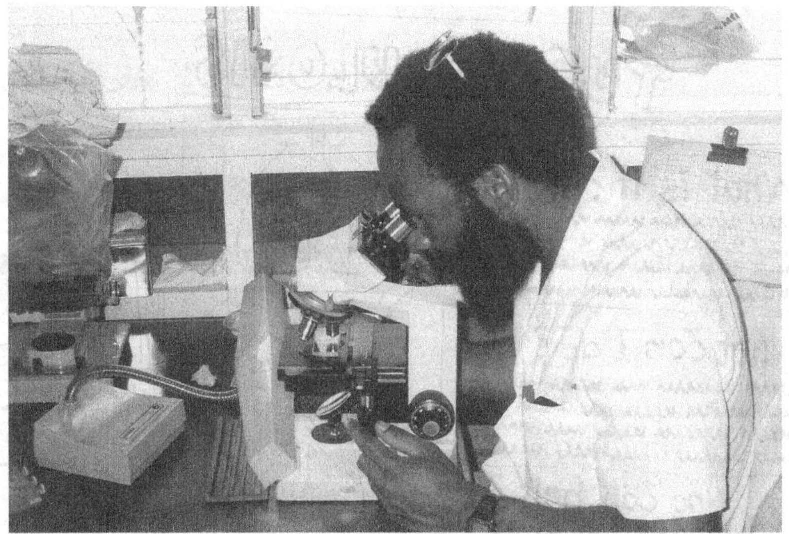

A lab worker at Telefomin Health Centre in West Sepik Province looking through a microscope.

INFORMATION

DOTS

- In 1998, the National Department of Health started a program called DOTS (Directly Observed Treatment Shortcourse).
- The DOTS program involves giving TB patients two weeks of education and treatment at a hospital.
- In most cases, the patient is sent home to complete a further six months of supervised treatment in close consultation with the hospital.

Activity 2·5 *Presenting a TB chart*

For this activity, you will be making an information display about TB. Use the information in this book and look for information in the library or from a health centre.

Include magazine and newspaper pictures, and health information booklets from health centres.

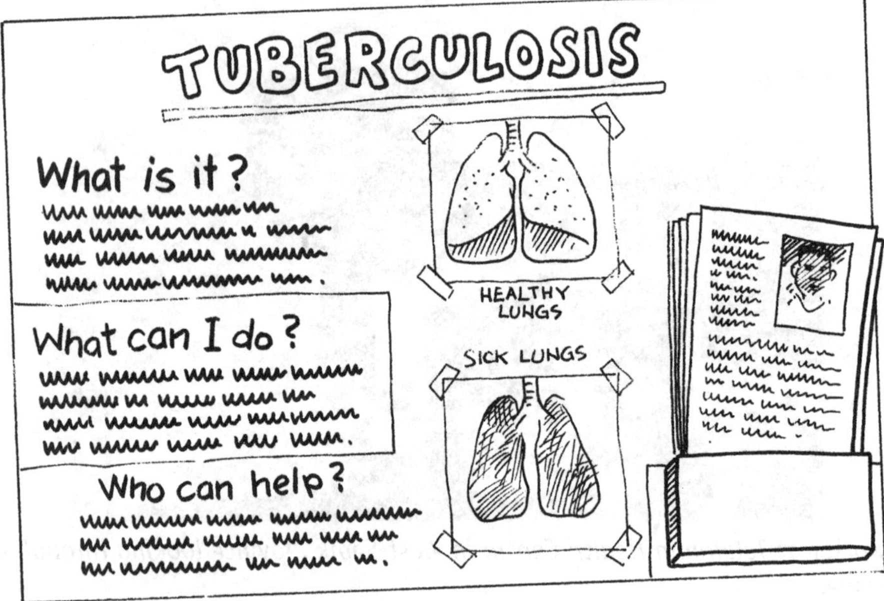

These are the basic questions your display should be able to answer:

- What is TB?
- How do you get TB?
- How can people keep from getting TB?
- What treatment is there for TB?
- Where should people go for a TB check-up?
- Which other diseases have symptoms like those of TB?
- How do you know whether you have TB?

Frank

The figure lay peacefully without moving. Relatives surrounded him; some just stared, while others tried to comfort his grieving wife. George had died from TB. Frank, his only son, stood under a tree looking at the people going to pay their last respects to the man he had loved so dearly all his life.

'Oh God, why did you have to take him away?' he thought aloud. 'If only I had known what to do about his sickness. I could have helped my father and he would be alive today.'

After the funeral, Frank decided that he would make a change by helping other people know more about TB. First, he went to the hospital where Dr Saun gave him information about the symptoms of TB.

'When people have TB they cough, they have chest pains, they get a fever and night sweats. They also lose weight quickly,' he said. 'It is a disease that is curable; it can be treated with medicine. But the treatment lasts six months, so sometimes it is difficult to make people take the whole treatment.'

Frank told Dr Saun that his father was treated for TB but that it had failed him and he died.

'It was probably too late to treat the sickness when we finally attended to him. Or perhaps he did not complete all his medicine,' said Doctor Saun. 'Let me explain to you about the DOTS system we use to treat TB patients.'

'What is DOTS?' Frank asked.

'DOTS is a chemotherapy treatment. After two months of daily treatment with four kinds of medicine, the saliva of a TB patient is checked again for TB germs,' said the doctor. 'If the patient appears to be getting better, he or she will be given two kinds of medicine twice a week for about four months. This means that the treatment lasts six months.'

Dr Saun also told Frank that the treatment can take eight or nine months if patients have already been cured of TB in the past but have become infected again. Sometimes the TB can get into other parts of the body.

'TB treatment must be completed even if the patient appears to have recovered,' said Dr Saun. 'Even though patients feel better and their symptoms go away, they should not stop taking their medicine. TB germs may still be in the body. They will be the strongest and most dangerous of

→

all the germs.'

Frank heard and understood all that the good doctor had told him. He remembered the good times he had with his father and vowed to cherish them in his mind.

'Although my father is gone, I will remember him and help to educate more people about this disease,' he said.

The doctor thought that if change was to happen in society, then men like Frank were the way to make people aware of the program.

'You are a brave young man,' said the doctor.

'I am more determined because I don't want to see other people die of TB like my father,' replied Frank.

Frank continued his drive to learn more about TB and never stopped striving in school either.

He helped in community awareness programs and became a good example to other youths in promoting TB prevention programs.

After reading Frank's story, answer the following questions.

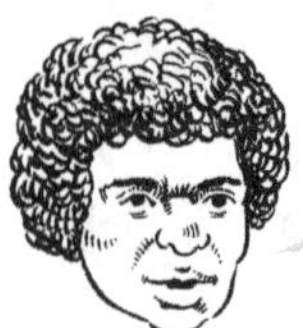

1. What disease did Franks father die of?
2. What do you think of Doctor Saun?
3. What is DOTS?
4. What is the treatment for TB?

Activity 3·3 *Miriam*

Miriam was told by her doctor that she had TB. She was told to take her medication for six months and to turn up for a review with the doctor. The doctor also gave her a schedule for medication and review.

Miriam took her medicine for a period of four months. But because she started to feel well, she decided to quit treatment and go to the village.

After six months Miriam felt sick and the TB symptoms began to show again. She returned to the hospital to find out what was wrong with her.

After reading about Miriam, answer the following questions:

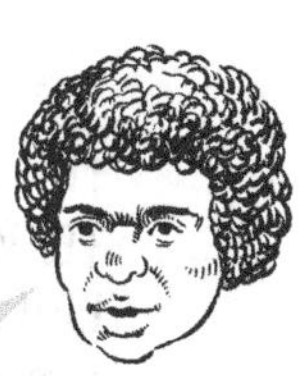

1 Why did Miriam start to feel sick again?
2 Do you think Miriam was right to stop her TB treatment before if was complete?
3 Why is it important to complete TB treatment?
4 What do you think the doctor said to Miriam when she showed up at the hospital?
5 If you were in Miriam's situation, what would you have done?

Questions and Answers

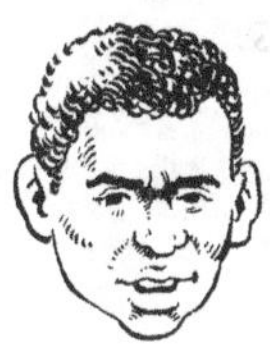

What happens if a person does not finish a TB treatment?

People will most likely get sick again if they do not complete the TB treatment. The next time, the medicine may not work.

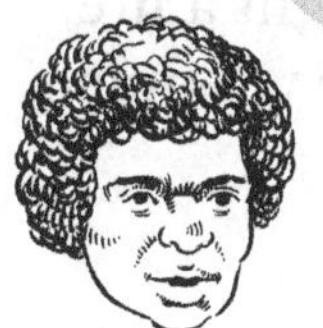

How can we stop the spread of TB?

Spitting, coughing and sneezing can spread TB very easily, so care should always be taken not to infect someone this way.

Using a handkerchief is an easy way to avoid infecting other people. If people have TB, it is important that they complete the full treatment.

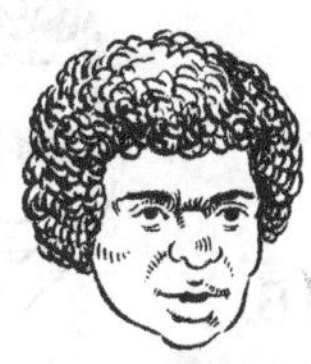

What should I do if I think a family member has TB?

Take the person to a health clinic for a check-up. The whole family should go to find out if the disease has spread.

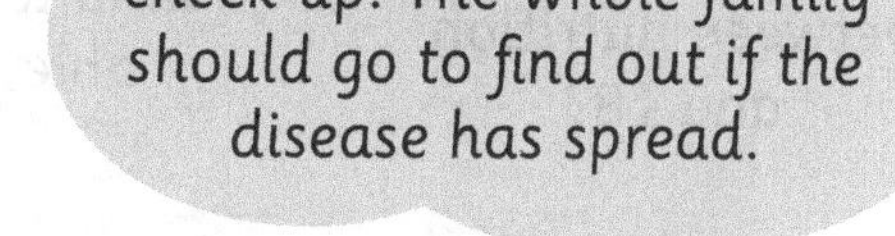

The only vaccine to prevent TB is the BCG vaccine. Unfortunately, this vaccine does not protect you completely. It should be given to all children to prevent dangerous forms of TB such as TB of the brain or TB that spreads to all organs. BCG is given at birth, school entry and school leaving.

Can TB be prevented?

TB can be prevented by medications, vaccinations, and by proper living and working conditions. But these will not totally prevent TB.

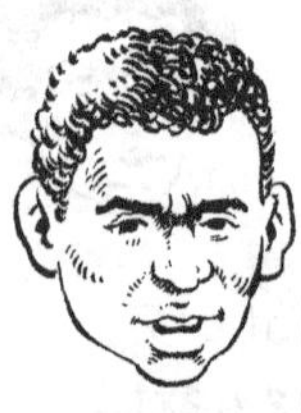

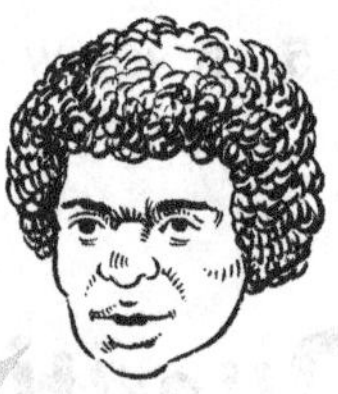

Anti-TB drugs must be given to children under five who have had contact with saliva from TB patients. This will stop the TB infection from developing.

The likelihood of breathing and contracting TB germs is much higher if you share a room with an infectious TB patient. The rooms of your house should have adequate light and good air flow. You should not light a fire in a closed room because smoke from the fire can damage your windpipe and lungs making it easier to get lung infections.

Is there any relation between nutrition and TB?

Yes.
Children who do not eat well have a greater chance of getting TB. Healthy food will keep the immune system strong and able to fight disease.

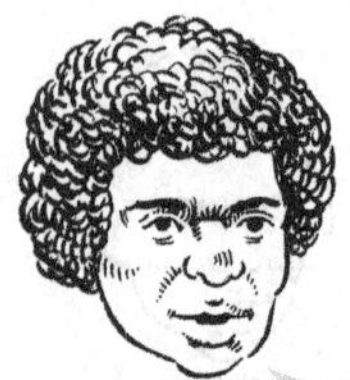

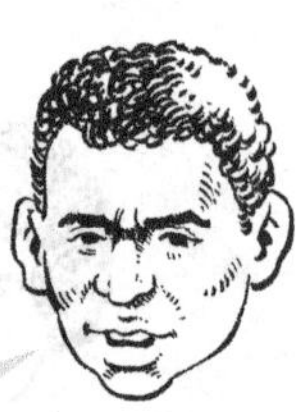

Chapter 4 Diarrhoea and vomiting – Gastrointestinal diseases

Diarrhoea and vomiting are very common symptoms of disease in the gastrointestinal system. Diarrhoea is one of the most common causes of death in children in Papua New Guinea.

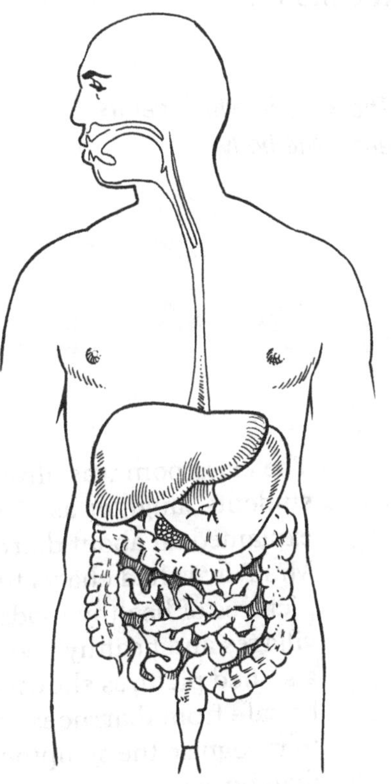
The gastrointestinal system

 Diarrhoea

Diarrhoea is watery faeces. Normal faeces is passed once or twice a day, but diarrhoea is passed many times over the day. This can cause dehydration (loss of body water).

There are three kinds of diarrhoea:

Acute watery diarrhoea

This is the most common kind of diarrhoea. Most deaths from acute watery diarrhoea are caused by dehydration. Patients are given lots of water (by mouth or by a tube into the body) to treat it.

Dysentery

Dysentery is faeces with blood in it. This is found in few cases but causes many deaths. Antibiotics and lots of water are used to treat this kind of diarrhoea.

Persistent diarrhoea

This is diarrhoea that lasts for more than 14 day. This is the least common kind of diarrhoea, but many people who get it die from it. It is usually caused by severe malnutrition. Intensive medical treatment is required.

What causes diarrhoea?

Diarrhoea has many causes but infection and malnutrition are the most important causes.

The most common ways germs cause diarrhoea is through them entering the mouth.

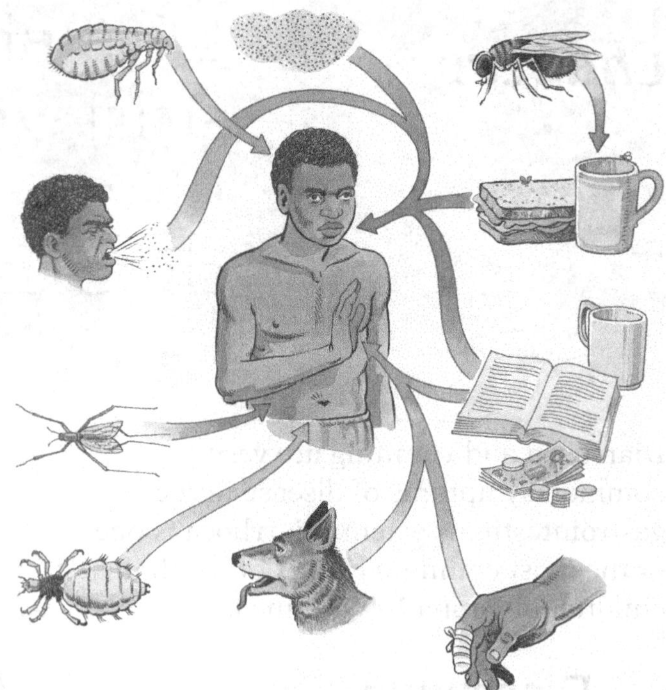

The ways in which germs enter the body.

Maria

The classroom was alive with the students' laughter as Mrs Petrus explained all about diarrhoea. Mrs Petrus had charts that had pictures of healthy foods, healthy villages and healthy people. Some also had pictures showing how to be safe from diarrhoea and how to recognise the symptoms of diarrhoea.

'People who have diarrhoea become dehydrated very quickly because their faeces is more loose and watery than usual. If untreated, diarrhoea can lead to death. Many children die from diarrhoea every year because they do not receive proper treatment soon enough. Malnourished children are most likely to get diarrhoea because their bodies are too weak to fight infections.'

Maria was sitting at the back of the class. She was anxious to know more about diarrhoea. She remembered the time when mother had to carry her to the hospital because she was so sick. She could still hear the nurse telling her mother that dirty hands and contaminated drinking water are the main causes of diarrhoea. The nurse said that germs that live in unclean places enter the mouth after they come in contact with food or water, cooking and eating utensils, or dirty hands during food preparation or feeding.

Mrs Petrus showed the class more pictures about diarrhoea and the class looked on with interest. 'The germs that enter through the mouth infect the intestine. This stops your body from using the water and nutrients when you eat. You will pass more faeces than usual. This means you will lose all of the things that you body needs—like water, vitamins and minerals.'

Maria let her mind drift off. She imagined germs floating to her, calling to her. Some germs were smiling and saying that they could become good friends if only she had dirty fingers and drank dirty water.

'I can stay in your body and be a good friend to you if only you let me come in!' said one of them.

'I can give you diarrhoea!' exclaimed a cheeky germ.

'We can be passed in the faeces so the infection can spread when people come into contact with us! We get to meet all sorts of people that way!' said a dirty germ who floated by Maria.

'Our friends, measles and pneumonia, can also give you diarrhoea,' said another little germ.

Maria heard the class roar with laughter and slowly opened her eyes to see that they were laughing at her. Malcolm, the big bully, was laughing so hard that Maria wished that he would have a heart attack and disappear forever.

'Well, that's enough laughing at Maria,' said Mrs Petrus. She told Maria that she could go and wash her face next time she felt sleepy.

Maria apologised and she promised that she would try to stay awake next time to learn more about diarrhoea and children.

She thought of the germs and vowed to tell her mother about diarrhoea and probably skip the sleeping part.

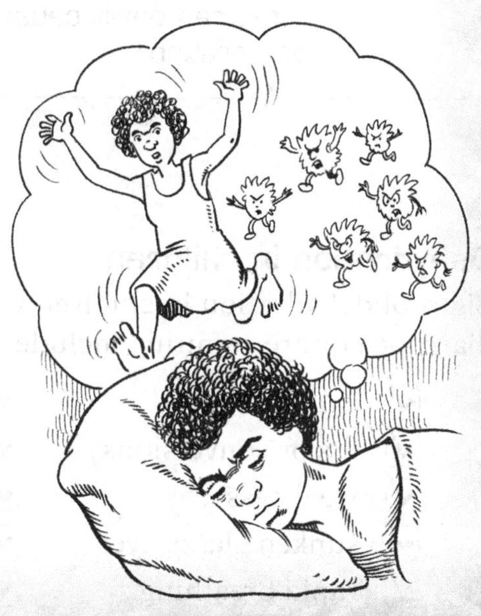

After reading Maria's story, answer the following questions.

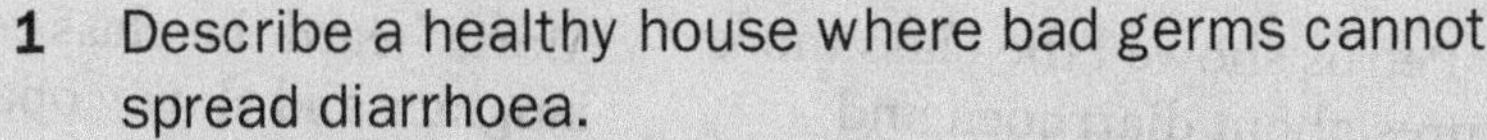

1 Describe a healthy house where bad germs cannot spread diarrhoea.

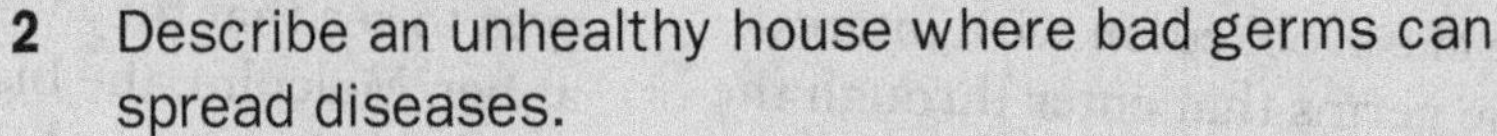

2 Describe an unhealthy house where bad germs can spread diseases.

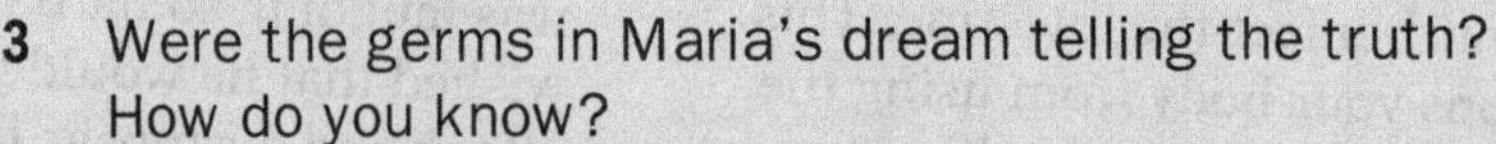

3 Were the germs in Maria's dream telling the truth? How do you know?

4 How can you keep germs that cause diarrhoea away from your school?

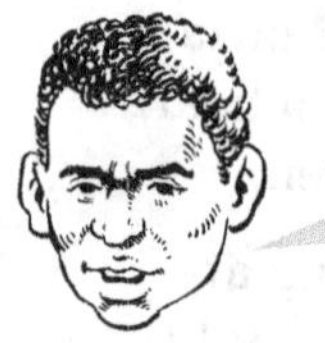

INFORMATION

Dehydration

- Dehydration is loss of body fluid.
- Loss of body fluids in diarrhoea faeces or vomit can easily cause dehydration.

Early treatment of diarrhoea usually prevents dehydration. People with diarrhoea usually get better quickly if they are given enough proper fluids to drink.

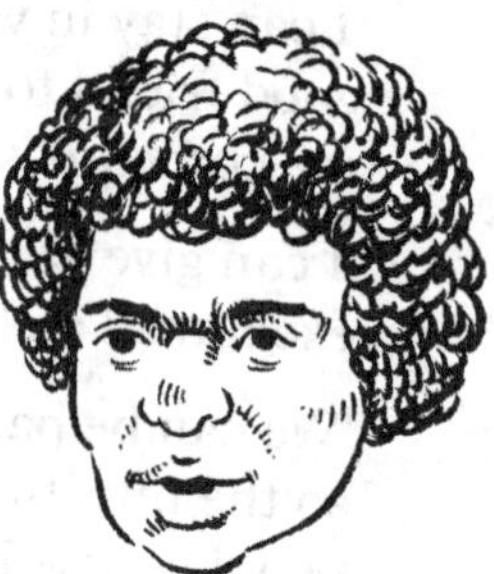

Dehydration in children

Signs of dehydration in children who have diarrhoea or are vomiting include:

- ☑ extreme thirst
- ☑ fits or convulsions
- ☑ weakness
- ☑ sunken glassy eyes
- ☑ rapid breathing
- ☑ rapid pulse
- ☑ dark-coloured urine
- ☑ little or no urine
- ☑ dry, loose skin
- ☑ sudden weight loss
- ☑ dry mouth, lips, tongue.

It is very important to drink fluids when diarrhoea begins. Ensure that children are given lots of water as soon as they have symptoms of diarrhoea.

How can diarrhoea be treated at home?

Children with mild diarrhoea can be treated at home. Proper foods and liquids should be provided.

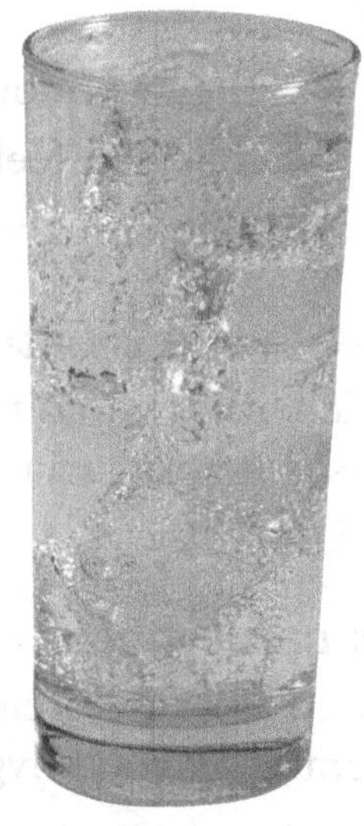

- ☑ Fresh fruit juices (pawpaw, guavas, oranges, or passion fruit are especially good for diarrhoea patients).
- ☑ Coconut water, rice water, sugar water, soup and weak tea will also put more fluid back into the body.

If children have severe diarrhoea, dehydration and other complications, they must be sent to the nearest health centre or hospital for emergency treatment. Go to the hospital immediately if the child's condition does not improve.

It is important to remember that children with diarrhoea must never be neglected.

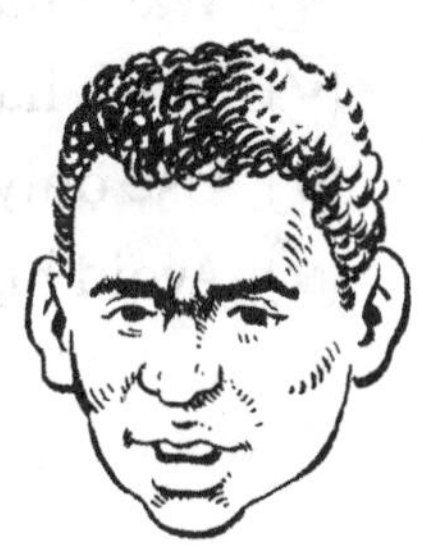

 Typhoid

Typhoid is an infectious bacterial fever that attacks the body's intestines. It generally occurs where there is bad sanitation and hygiene. The germ can get into food and into the water supply through poor hygiene and sanitation. It is spread from person to person through faeces.

Typhoid bacteria can live for months or years in the bodies of people who have recovered from typhoid infection. These people are called carriers of the infection. Carriers pass the typhoid germs out of the body through faeces and urine.

What are the symptoms of typhoid?

It takes about 10 to 14 days for the germs to multiply and cause symptoms. During this time the person may not have any definite symptoms and just feel unwell. At the end of the second week the person may complain of severe abdominal pain, diarrhoea and a bad cough.

It is difficult to diagnose typhoid fever. Typhoid should be suspected when:

- the fever does not decrease after malaria treatment
- a person feels unwell and is first constipated, then has diarrhoea
- a person has diarrhoea and a tender abdomen.

What is the treatment for typhoid?

People with typhoid must visit a health centre for a malaria test. If the illness is not malaria then a course of the proper antibiotics is needed to treat typhoid.

How can typhoid be prevented?

Typhoid fever is spread by poor hygiene. This means that it can be prevented by good hygiene:

- Only use good toilets built in the right place.
- Wash hands thoroughly after going to the toilet.
- Wash hands before cooking and eating.
- Use only clean safe drinking water.
- Avoid buying food and water from unhygienic places.

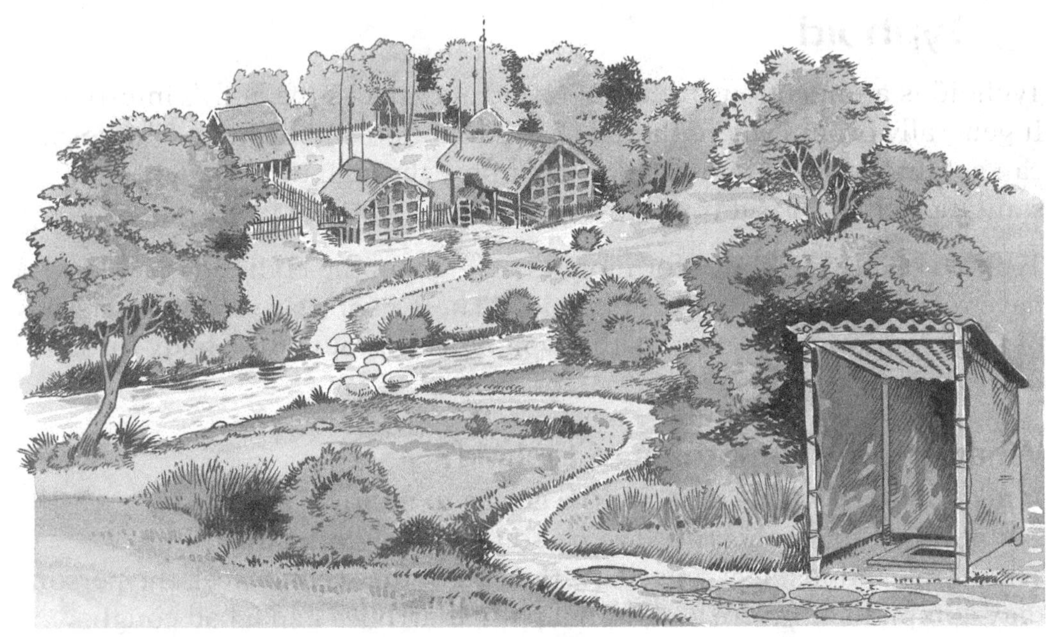

Chapter 5 Sores and skin diseases

Some skin diseases, such as scabies and ringworm, harm only the skin while the rest of the body is healthy. Other skin diseases, such as measles and leprosy, cause lesions (abnormal parts) inside the body as well as on the skin. Usually in these illnesses the lesions inside the body are more dangerous.

Most of the skin diseases that harm only the person's skin are due to germs getting onto the skin. The germs multiply there if they are not washed off with soap and water.

Cleanliness is very important when you have skin diseases. Cleaning the skin and wounds will prevent infection.

Scabies

Scabies is a very common skin problem. It is caused by a small insect that burrows holes into the skin. Scabies is not a dangerous illness but it causes lots of unhappiness. The sores it causes are itchy. This makes people uncomfortable because they have to scratch a lot and have trouble sleeping and eating.

Scabies are very small insects. This is what one looks like magnified.

What are the symptoms of scabies?

- ☑ itchy rash often between fingers and on buttocks, genitals and abdomen
- ☑ raised lesions, sometimes with pus in them.

What is the treatment for scabies?

Scabies lotion is painted on the skin to kill the scabies insects. All parts of the body must be painted except the face. All family members should be treated at the same time.

Because scabies spread easily from person to person, it is important that the entire family be treated.

The following steps should be taken:

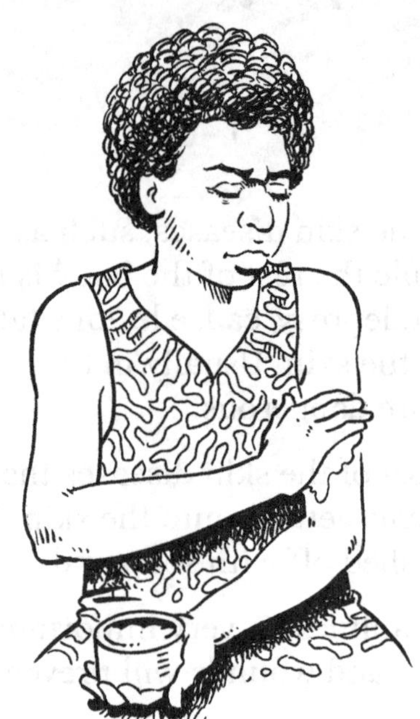

- ☑ All family members must wash their entire bodies with soap and water.
- ☑ The lotion must be painted on the entire body, except the face.
- ☑ All dirty clothes, blankets and mats must be washed.
- ☑ Washed clothing, blankets and mats must be put in the sun to dry to kill the insects.
- ☑ The lotion must be washed off after 24 hours.
- ☑ The entire process must be repeated four days later.

 Chicken pox

Chicken pox is a disease that causes a high fever, itchy blisters and a rash all over the body. Scratching the rash can result in scarring.

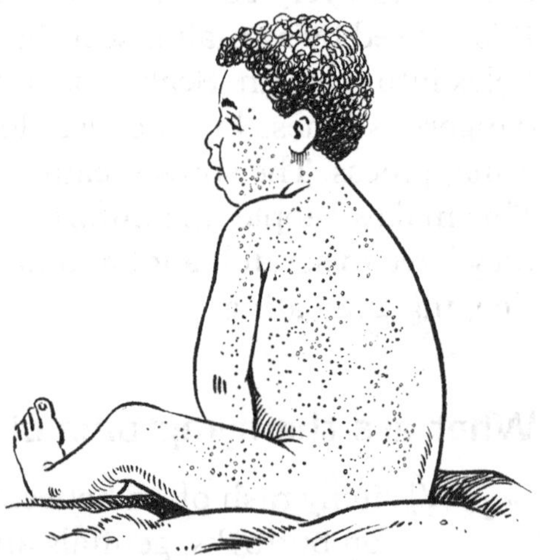

What are the symptoms of chicken pox?

- ☑ fever
- ☑ loss of appetite
- ☑ rash
- ☑ small blisters all over the body.

What is the treatment for chicken pox?

- ☑ The entire body must be washed with soap and water.
- ☑ If sores become infected, you should get antibiotic treatment at a clinic or health centre.
- ☑ If there is any pain, take paracetamol.

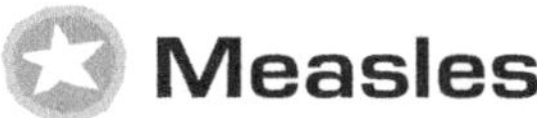

Measles

Measles is a very infectious viral disease passed to others by coughing and sneezing. It takes 14 days to get sick after you have been infected. It may affect children of any age.

What are the symptoms of measles?

- fever
- running nose
- sore eyes
- rash (after two days).

What is the treatment for measles?

- Use paracetamol for fever.
- Wash body regularly to lessen itching.

How can measles be prevented?

Measles can be prevented with immunisation.

Boils and abscesses

Boils and abscesses are skin infections that cause pus to collect under the skin.

A boil starts as an infection in the hair follicle (the part of the hair under the skin). It is a round hard swelling and is always tender and usually has a small head on it. It always bursts by itself.

An abscess is a large, pus-filled lesion under the skin. It sometimes gets into the muscles.

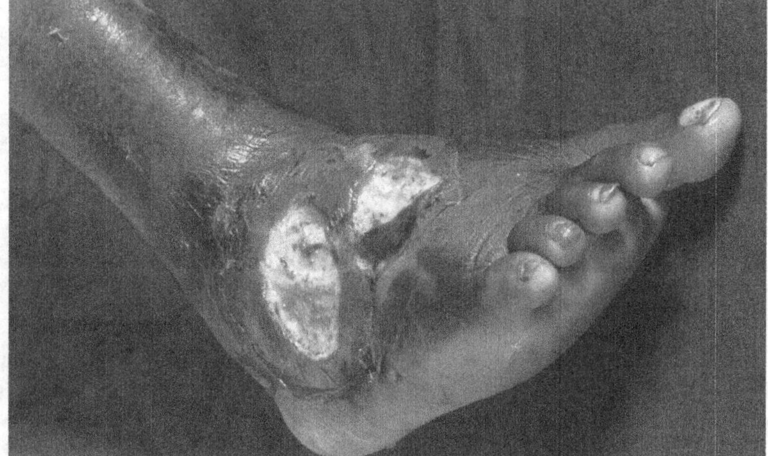

What is the treatment for boils?

Keep the wound clean.

What is the treatment for abscesses?

If pus is present in an abscess it must be cut at the Aid Post or health centre so that the pus can be drained.

Antibiotics should be taken to prevent further infection.

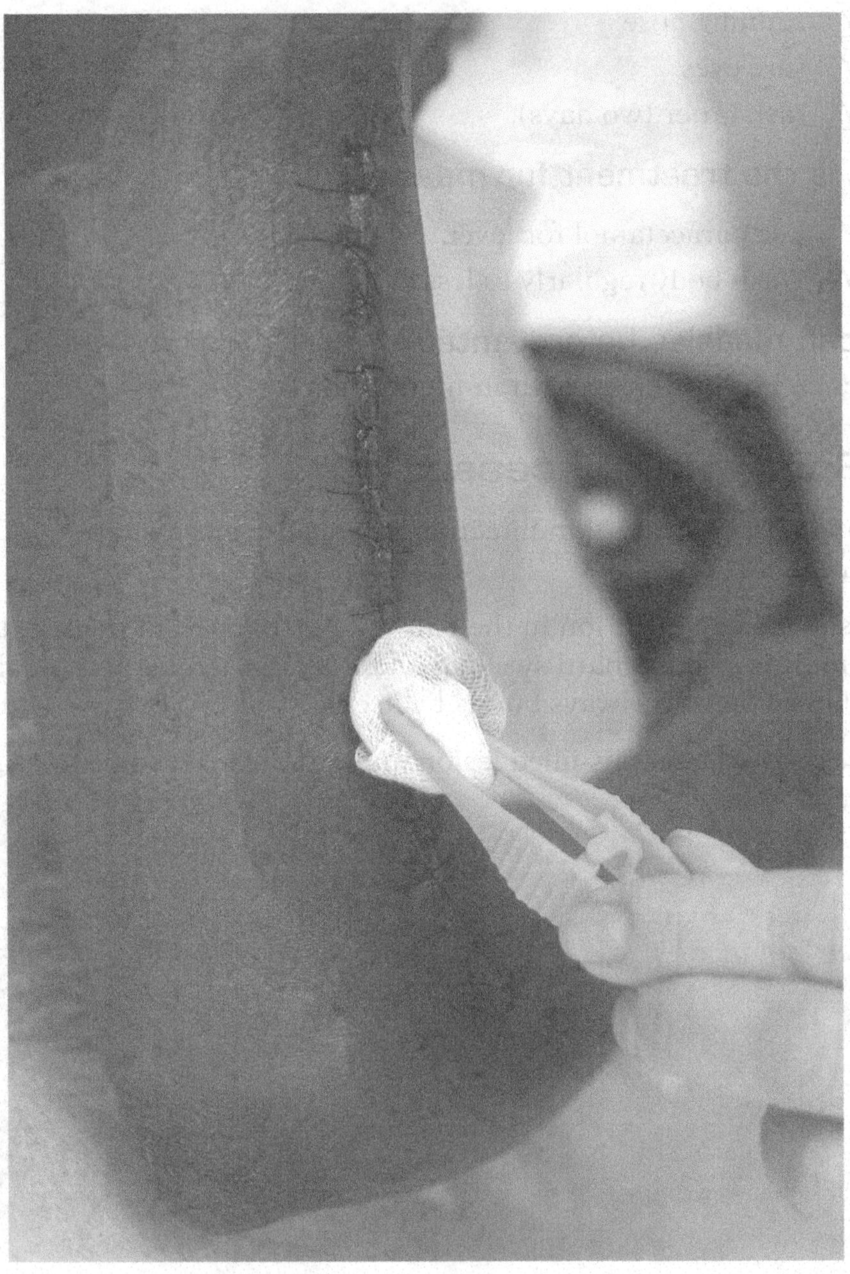

Chapter 6 Food and nutritional diseases

Malnutrition means 'bad nutrition'. It is caused by a poor diet or by the body's inability to absorb or use nutrients.

Malnutrition is very common in Papua New Guinea. Malnourished children get infections easily and die more easily than other children.

Primary malnutrition results when the body:

- ☑ gets too much food
  or
- ☑ does not get enough food
  or
- ☑ gets the wrong kinds of food.

When people are already sick, secondary malnutrition may result. The body cannot use the nutrients that people eat even though they are present in the food. This happens when a person has diarrhoea or typhoid, for example.

People can also suffer from malnutrition when environmental conditions are not good. Natural disasters, like flooding and drought, cause disruptions in food supply and can make drinking water unsafe.

Ignorance about good food choices can also cause malnutrition. Eating food that is good for you is an important part of avoiding malnutrition.

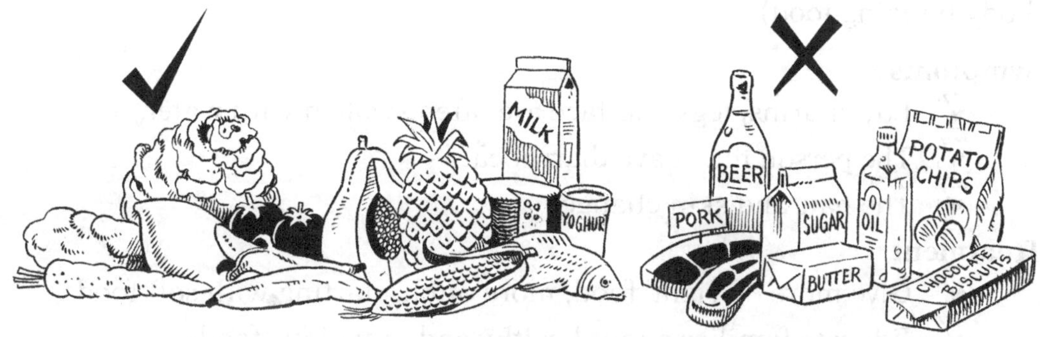

Obesity and starvation are extreme forms of malnutrition.

When people eat much more food than they need, or they eat the wrong kinds of food (like too much fat or sugar), they can become obese.

Starvation is under-nourishment. When people do not eat enough food, they will suffer from under-nourishment. People who are undernourished can lose weight and become weak. They may also have diarrhoea and cramps.

 Protein-energy malnutrition

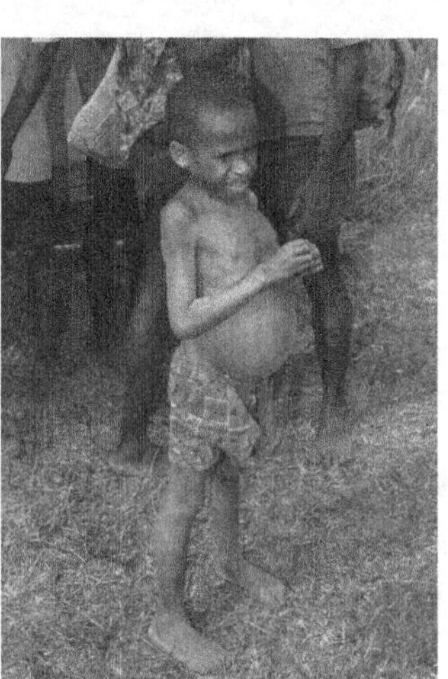

This child has marasmus.

Marasmus

This type of malnutrition occurs when the diet is very low in proteins and calories. A child with marasmus has eaten so little protein and energy food that the child is very underweight (weighs less than 60 per cent of the average weight).

Symptoms

- ☑ The person weighs less than 60 per cent of the average weight.
- ☑ Muscle and fat waste away. This may make a child look very old.
- ☑ The person may have diarrhoea and anaemia.

Treatment

- ☑ Give more of 'right' food, more often, starting with soft food.
- ☑ Educate families about healthy and nutritious foods.

Kwashiorkor

Kwashiorkor occurs in children who have not eaten enough protein (body-building food).

Symptoms

- ☑ Lower arms, legs and face are often swollen with water.
- ☑ The person may have diarrhoea.
- ☑ The hair and skin change.

Treatment

- ☑ Give more of 'right' food, more often, starting with soft food.
- ☑ Educate families about healthy and nutritious foods.

Overweight from eating too much

Being overweight can cause problems such as heart disease and joint disease. Adults and children who do not exercise enough or who eat too much can become overweight.

People who are overweight should eat less than they usually do. They should not starve themselves, however. It is important that a reasonable amount of healthy food—such as fresh fruits, vegetables, and lean meat—be eaten every day. Packaged food and snack foods should be avoided.

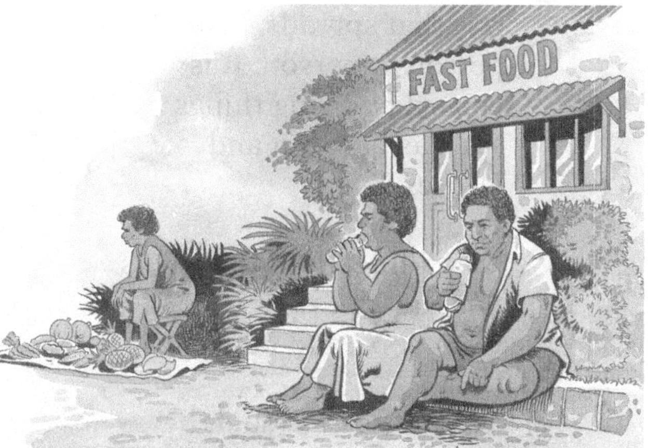

Many of the foods we need can be grown in Papua New Guinea. People in villages grow most of their food but those in towns or growing cash crops may buy most of their food in markets or shops. People in towns must realise that it is important to buy the right kinds of foods and enough food to have a balanced diet. Careful shopping and planning is needed to find the cheapest source of a balanced diet.

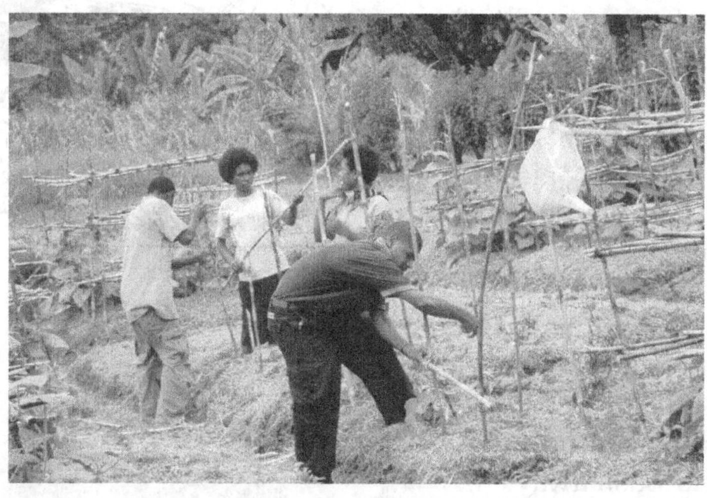

People can grow healthy food in their own or community gardens.

What have we learnt?

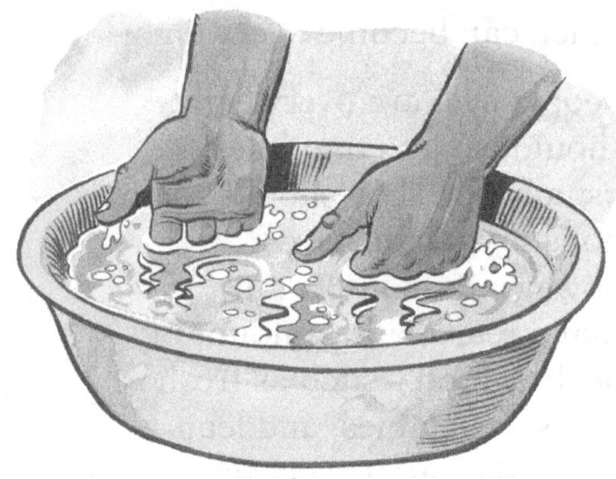

- ☑ An infectious disease is one that spreads from person to person. It is caused by living things such as bacteria and viruses.
- ☑ A non-infectious disease is one that does not spread from person to person.
- ☑ Many diseases (such as measles, whooping cough, diphtheria and polio) can be prevented by immunisation or vaccination.

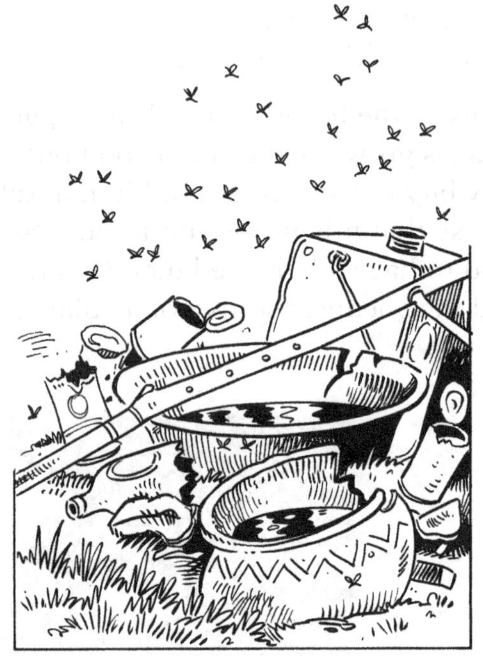

- ☑ The main features of malaria are fever and chills, headache, tiredness, anaemia, large spleen.
- ☑ Patients with severe malaria may also vomit, have fits and be unable to stand.
- ☑ To prevent malaria people need to get rid of breeding places for mosquitoes, clear bush away from houses and use treated mosquito nets.

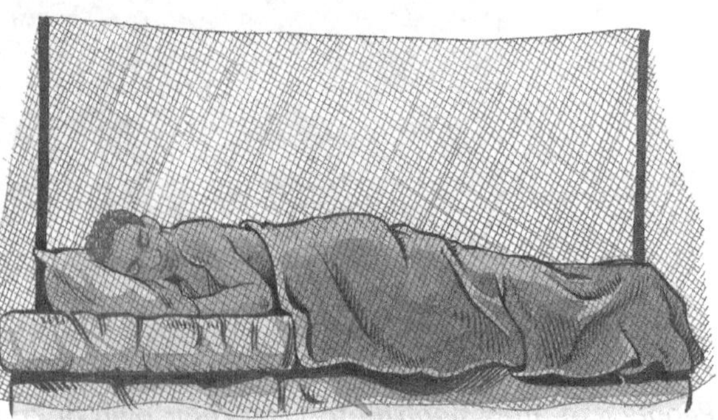

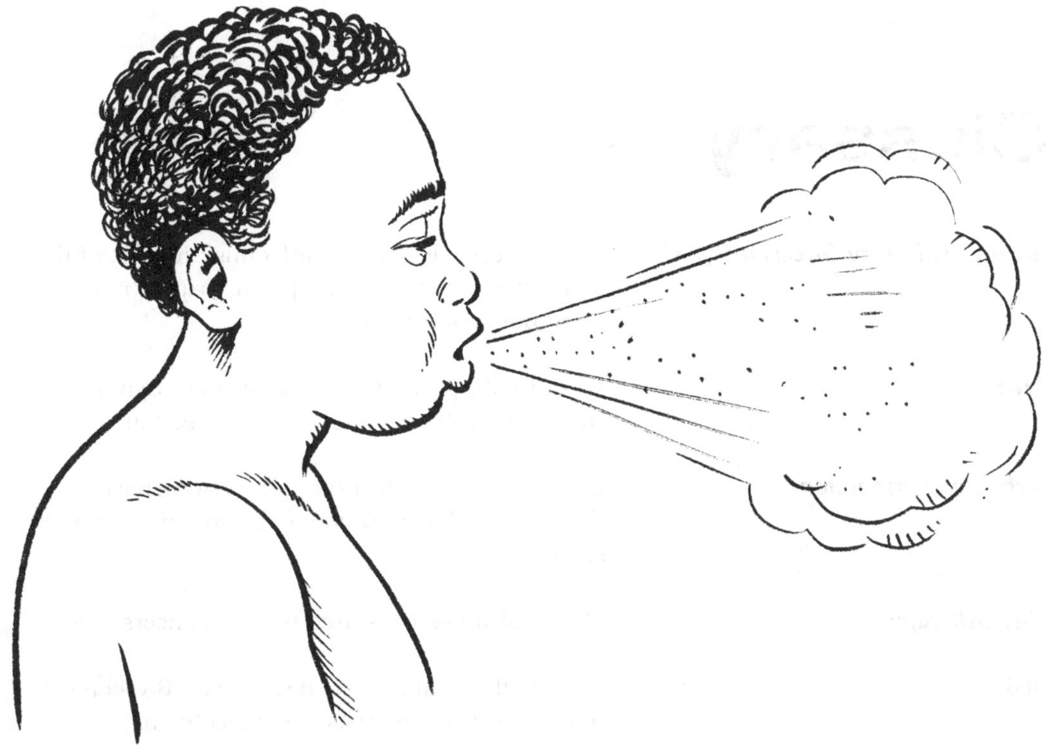

- ☑ ARIs (acute respiratory infections) are infections of the lungs and breathing passages. Serious ARIs include pneumonia, whooping cough and TB, which can cause death. Other common ARIs include the common cold, tonsillitis, laryngitis and bronchitis.
- ☑ Malnutrition is a serious problem that is common in Papua New Guinea. Malnutrition is caused by lack of food or lack of the right kind of food. Malnutrition makes infections worse.
- ☑ Anything abnormal on the skin is called a skin lesion.

Glossary

Acute Respiratory Infections (ARI)	acute infectious diseases affecting any part of the respiratory tract; for example, flu, runny nose, pneumonia and the like
AIDS	short for Acquired Immunodeficiency Syndrome; the terminal (final) stage of HIV infection
airborne transmission	transmission of infectious germs by airborne droplets produced by coughing, sneezing, and speaking
chemotherapy	chemical substances used to treat cancers
BCG	the Bacillius Calmette and Gourine TB vaccine, named for the scientists who invented it
fever	a rise in body temperature making the body feel hot and sweaty, and the pulse to go faster; comes with many illnesses, especially malaria, measles and typhoid
germ	any micro-organism (for instance bacterium, virus protozoan), especially one that causes disease
HIV	short for Human Immunodifficiency Virus, a disease that makes the human immune system break down and become more easily infected with other diseases
immune system	the body's defence system, which provides some protection against disease-causing germs
infection	invasion of the body by harmful germs
infectious	able to transmit germs to another person
microscope	a device used to see germs that cannot be seen with the naked eye

parasite	a small animal that lives on another animal
pneumonia	a dangerous respiratory infection affecting lungs
protozoa (singular: protozoon)	single-celled, microscopic living things
respiratory tract	the organs necessary for breathing: nose, middle ear, throat, voice box (larynx), windpipe (trachea), air passages (bronchi and bronchioles) and lungs
respiratory infection	an infection in any area of the respiratory tract
sputum	the mucus in spit after coughing
symptom	an indication of a disease or disorder noticed by the patient
syndrome	a combination of signs and / or symptoms that forms a distinct clinical picture indicative of a particular disorder
tuberculosis (TB)	chronic disease transmitted by airborne transmission caused by Mycobacterium tuberculosis
vaccine	a small injection of liquid to prevent infections
X-ray	a machine to take pictures of the inside of the body